Diabetic Diet

Cookbook for Beginners

2024

A Comprehensive Guide to Manage Diabetes with 4-Weeks Meal Plans and Tasty Recipes for Pre-Diabetes and Type 2 Diabetes, Featuring Low-Sugar and Low-Carbs Options

Rose B. Bright

Copyright © Rose B Bright 2024

Table of Contents

About the Author

With a passion for promoting healthy living through nutrition, **Rose B. Bright** is a renowned expert in the field of health-related diet cookbooks. Armed with extensive training and numerous accolades, she has dedicated her career to crafting culinary creations that nourish both the body and soul.

Rose B. Bright has garnered widespread recognition for her innovative approach to cooking, earning her a plethora of prestigious awards in the culinary world. Her recipes not only prioritize health and wellness but also tantalize taste buds with their exquisite flavors and textures.

Beyond her culinary expertise, Rose is a devoted advocate for balanced living, believing that a harmonious combination of wholesome food, regular exercise, and mindfulness is the key to overall well-being. Her commitment to this holistic approach shines through in her cookbooks, inspiring readers to embrace a lifestyle centered around health and vitality.

Outside of her professional pursuits, Rose finds joy and fulfillment in her role as a loving spouse. Her personal experiences infuse her writing with warmth and authenticity, making her cookbooks not only informative guides but also heartfelt reflections of her journey toward optimal health.

Through her work, Rose B. Bright empowers readers to take charge of their health and embark on a transformative culinary adventure. With each recipe meticulously crafted to enhance both physical health and culinary delight, she invites readers to join her on a flavorful journey toward a happier, healthier life."

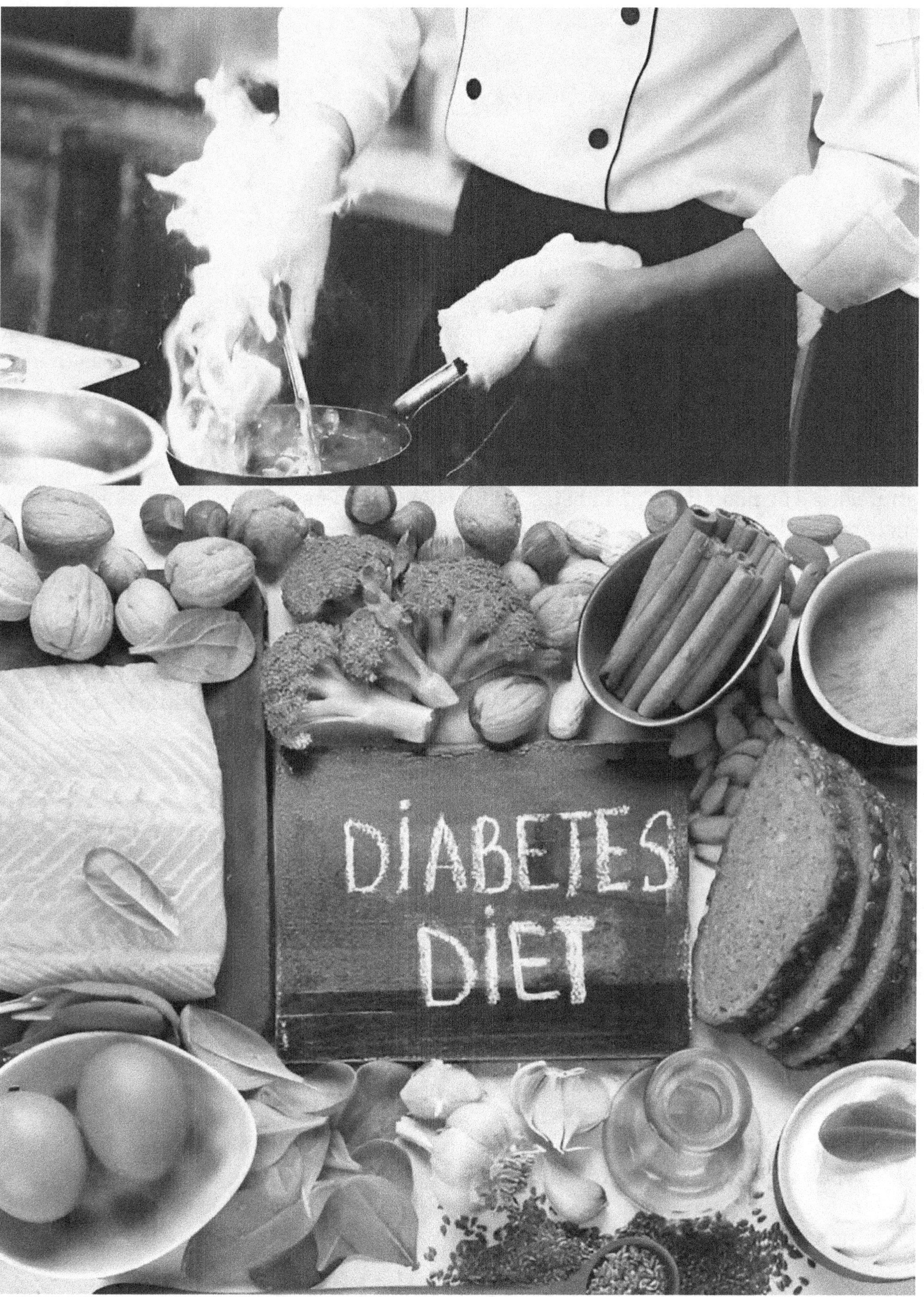
DIABETES
DIET

INTRODUCTION TO DIABETES AND HEALTHY EATING

Understanding Diabetes: Types, Symptoms, and Management

Diabetes is a chronic medical condition characterized by high levels of glucose (sugar) in the blood. It occurs when the body either does not produce enough insulin or cannot effectively use the insulin it produces. Insulin is a hormone produced by the pancreas that helps regulate blood sugar levels and allows glucose to enter the cells to be used as energy. Without enough insulin or if the body becomes resistant to insulin, glucose builds up in the bloodstream, leading to various health complications.

There are several types of diabetes, each with its own causes, symptoms, and management strategies. The main types of diabetes include type 1 diabetes, type 2 diabetes, gestational diabetes, and prediabetes.

1. Type 1 Diabetes:

Type 1 diabetes, also known as insulin-dependent diabetes or juvenile diabetes, is an autoimmune condition in which the immune system mistakenly attacks and destroys the insulin-producing cells in the pancreas. As a result, the body produces little to no insulin, leading to high blood sugar levels.

Symptoms of Type 1 Diabetes:-

- Excessive thirst
- Frequent urination
- Extreme hunger
- Unintended weight loss
- Fatigue and weakness
- Blurred vision
- Irritability and mood changes

Management of Type 1 Diabetes:-

The primary treatment for type 1 diabetes is insulin therapy, which involves regular injections of insulin to replace the hormone that the body cannot produce. Individuals with type 1 diabetes also need to monitor their blood sugar levels regularly, eat a balanced diet, engage in regular physical activity, and maintain a healthy lifestyle to manage their condition effectively.

2. Type 2 Diabetes:-

Type 2 diabetes is the most common form of diabetes, accounting for approximately 90-95% of all diagnosed cases. It occurs when the body becomes resistant to insulin or does not produce enough insulin to meet its needs. Type 2 diabetes is often associated with lifestyle factors such as obesity, unhealthy diet, lack of physical activity, and genetics.

Symptoms of Type 2 Diabetes:-

- Increased thirst and urination
- Fatigue
- Blurred vision
- Slow healing of wounds
- Tingling or numbness in the hands or feet
- Recurrent infections
- Darkened skin patches (acanthosis nigricans)

Management of Type 2 Diabetes:

The management of type 2 diabetes focuses on lifestyle modifications, including dietary changes, regular physical activity, weight management, and medication or insulin therapy if necessary. Diet plays a crucial role in managing type 2 diabetes, and individuals are often advised to follow a balanced diet that is low in refined sugars, saturated fats, and processed foods, and high in fiber-rich fruits, vegetables, whole grains, lean proteins, and healthy fats.

3. Gestational Diabetes:-

Gestational diabetes is a type of diabetes that develops during pregnancy, usually in the second or third trimester. It occurs when the body cannot produce enough insulin to meet the increased insulin needs during pregnancy. Gestational diabetes can increase the risk of complications during pregnancy and delivery if not properly managed.

Symptoms of Gestational Diabetes:-

Gestational diabetes often does not cause any noticeable symptoms. However, some women may experience symptoms such as:

- Increased thirst and urination
- Fatigue
- Blurred vision
- Recurrent infections

Management of Gestational Diabetes:-

The management of gestational diabetes typically involves dietary changes, regular physical activity, and blood sugar monitoring. In some cases, insulin therapy or medication may be necessary to help control blood sugar levels. It is essential for pregnant women with gestational diabetes to work closely with their healthcare team to ensure optimal management of their condition and reduce the risk of complications for both the mother and baby.

4. **Prediabetes**:-

Prediabetes is a condition in which blood sugar levels are higher than normal but not high enough to be diagnosed as type 2 diabetes. It is considered a precursor to type 2 diabetes and provides an opportunity for early intervention to prevent or delay the onset of diabetes.

Symptoms of Prediabetes:-

Prediabetes often does not cause any noticeable symptoms. However, some individuals may experience symptoms similar to those of type 2 diabetes, such as increased thirst and urination, fatigue, and blurred vision.

Management of Prediabetes:-

The management of prediabetes focuses on lifestyle modifications, including dietary changes, regular physical activity, and weight management. Making healthy lifestyle choices can help improve insulin sensitivity, lower blood sugar levels, and reduce the risk of developing type 2 diabetes.

In conclusion, understanding the types, symptoms, and management strategies of diabetes is crucial for individuals affected by this chronic condition and their healthcare providers. By learning about the different types of diabetes, recognizing the symptoms, and implementing effective management strategies, individuals can take control of their health and improve their quality of life. It is essential for individuals with diabetes to work closely with their healthcare team to develop a personalized treatment plan that addresses their specific needs and goals. Through education, awareness, and proactive management, individuals with diabetes can lead healthy, fulfilling lives while effectively managing their condition.

Importance of Diet in Diabetes Management

Diet plays a crucial role in the management of diabetes, a chronic metabolic disorder characterized by elevated blood sugar levels. For individuals with diabetes, making healthy food choices is essential for controlling blood sugar levels, preventing complications, and maintaining overall health and well-being. In this comprehensive discussion, we will explore the importance of diet in diabetes management, including the principles of a diabetes-friendly diet, the impact of dietary choices on blood sugar control, and practical tips for meal planning and healthy eating.

Impact of Dietary Choices on Blood Sugar Control

Dietary choices have a direct impact on blood sugar control in individuals with diabetes. By making informed food choices and adopting a balanced diet, individuals can effectively manage their blood sugar levels and reduce the risk of hyperglycemia (high blood sugar) and hypoglycemia (low blood sugar). Here are some ways in which dietary choices affect blood sugar control:

1. **Carbohydrate Content:**
   Monitoring carbohydrate intake and choosing foods with a lower glycemic index can help prevent spikes in blood sugar levels after meals. By balancing carbohydrate intake with protein, fiber, and healthy fats, individuals can achieve better blood sugar control throughout the day.

2. **Meal Timing and Portion Control:**
   Eating regular meals and snacks at consistent times can help stabilize blood sugar levels and prevent fluctuations. Portion control is also important to avoid overeating and maintain steady energy levels. By spreading carbohydrate intake evenly throughout the day and controlling portion sizes, individuals can prevent blood sugar spikes and crashes.

3. **Glycemic Index:**
   The glycemic index (GI) ranks carbohydrate-containing foods based on their effect on blood sugar levels. Foods with a low GI, such as whole grains, fruits, and vegetables, are digested more slowly and cause a gradual rise in blood sugar levels, while foods with a high GI, such as white bread, sugary snacks, and processed foods, cause rapid spikes in blood sugar levels. Choosing foods with a lower GI can help maintain stable blood sugar levels and improve overall glycemic control.

4. **Balance of Macronutrients:**
   Balancing the intake of carbohydrates, protein, and fats is essential for managing blood sugar levels and promoting satiety. Including lean protein sources and healthy fats in meals and snacks can help stabilize blood sugar levels, reduce hunger, and prevent overeating. Additionally, incorporating fiber-rich foods can slow down the absorption of glucose and improve blood sugar control.

BASICS OF A DIABETES-FRIENDLY DIET

A diabetes-friendly diet is a crucial component of managing diabetes effectively. It focuses on making healthy food choices to regulate blood sugar levels, prevent complications, and improve overall health and well-being. In this detailed discussion, we will explore the basics of a diabetes-friendly diet, including the principles of healthy eating, recommended food groups, portion control, and practical tips for meal planning.

Principles of a Diabetes-Friendly Diet

1. **Carbohydrate Control:** Carbohydrates have the most significant impact on blood sugar levels, making carbohydrate control a cornerstone of diabetes management. The goal is to manage the amount and type of carbohydrates consumed to prevent spikes in blood sugar levels. It involves choosing complex carbohydrates with a low glycemic index, such as whole grains, legumes, fruits, and vegetables, and monitoring portion sizes to avoid excessive carbohydrate intake.

2. **Emphasis on Fiber-Rich Foods:** Fiber is an essential nutrient for individuals with diabetes as it helps regulate blood sugar levels, improve digestion, and promote satiety. Including fiber-rich foods such as whole grains, fruits, vegetables, legumes, and nuts in the diet can help stabilize blood sugar levels and reduce the risk of heart disease. Aim to incorporate a variety of fiber-rich foods into meals and snacks to maximize their health benefits.

3. **Lean Protein Sources:** Protein is important for maintaining muscle mass, regulating blood sugar levels, and promoting satiety. Lean protein sources such as poultry, fish, tofu, legumes, and low-fat dairy products are recommended for individuals with diabetes. Including protein in meals and snacks can help stabilize blood sugar levels, prevent overeating, and support overall health.

4. **Healthy Fats:** Healthy fats play a crucial role in diabetes management by improving insulin sensitivity, lowering inflammation, and reducing the risk of heart disease. Sources of healthy fats include avocados, nuts, seeds, olive oil, and fatty fish. It is important to consume these fats in moderation and avoid sources of saturated and trans fats, which can increase the risk of heart disease.

5. **Limitation of Sugary and Processed Foods:** Sugary and processed foods should be limited in a diabetes-friendly diet due to their high carbohydrate and calorie content. These foods can cause rapid spikes in blood sugar levels and

contribute to weight gain, insulin resistance, and increased risk of complications. Instead, focus on whole, unprocessed foods and choose natural sweeteners such as stevia or monk fruit when needed.

Recommended Food Groups

1. **Non-Starchy Vegetables:** Non-starchy vegetables are low in carbohydrates and calories, making them an excellent choice for individuals with diabetes. These include leafy greens, broccoli, cauliflower, bell peppers, cucumbers, tomatoes, and zucchini. Non-starchy vegetables are high in fiber, vitamins, minerals, and antioxidants, making them an important part of a diabetes-friendly diet.

2. **Whole Grains:** Whole grains are rich in fiber, vitamins, minerals, and antioxidants, making them a nutritious choice for individuals with diabetes. Examples of whole grains include brown rice, quinoa, barley, oats, whole wheat bread, and whole grain pasta. Choose whole grains over refined grains whenever possible to maximize their health benefits.

3. **Lean Proteins:** Lean protein sources are important for maintaining muscle mass, regulating blood sugar levels, and promoting satiety. Include lean protein sources such as poultry, fish, tofu, legumes, and low-fat dairy products in meals and snacks. Avoid processed meats and choose lean cuts of meat to reduce saturated fat intake.

4. **Healthy Fats:** Healthy fats are beneficial for individuals with diabetes as they help improve insulin sensitivity, lower inflammation, and reduce the risk of heart disease. Include sources of healthy fats such as avocados, nuts, seeds, olive oil, and fatty fish in the diet. Limit saturated and trans fats found in processed and fried foods to reduce the risk of heart disease.

5. **Fruits:** Fruits are nutritious and provide essential vitamins, minerals, and antioxidants. While fruits contain natural sugars, they can be included in moderation as part of a balanced diet for individuals with diabetes. Choose whole fruits over fruit juices and dried fruits, which are higher in sugar and lower in fiber.

Portion Control:

Portion control is an important aspect of managing diabetes and controlling blood sugar levels. It involves monitoring portion sizes to avoid overeating and consuming excessive calories and carbohydrates. Some practical tips for portion control include:

- Use smaller plates and bowls to control portion sizes.
- Measure serving sizes using measuring cups, spoons, or a food scale.
- Pay attention to recommended serving sizes on food labels.
- Fill half of your plate with non-starchy vegetables, one-quarter with lean protein, and one-quarter with whole grains or starchy vegetables.
- Be mindful of portion sizes when eating out or ordering takeout.

Practical Tips for Meal Planning

1. **Plan Ahead:** Plan meals and snacks in advance to ensure a balanced and nutritious diet. Consider factors such as carbohydrate content, protein sources, and portion sizes when planning meals.
2. **Prepare Meals at Home:** Cooking meals at home allows you to control ingredients and portion sizes, making it easier to follow a diabetes-friendly diet. Experiment with healthy recipes and cooking methods to add variety to your meals.
3. **Include a Variety of Foods:** Incorporate a variety of foods from different food groups into your meals to ensure a balanced diet. Experiment with different fruits, vegetables, whole grains, lean proteins, and healthy fats to add flavor and nutrition to your meals.
4. **Monitor Blood Sugar Levels:** Monitor your blood sugar levels regularly to assess the impact of dietary choices on your blood sugar control. Keep track of your carbohydrate intake and how different foods affect your blood sugar levels to make informed decisions about your diet.
5. **Seek Support:** Seek support from a registered dietitian or certified diabetes educator to develop a personalized meal plan that meets your nutritional needs and lifestyle.

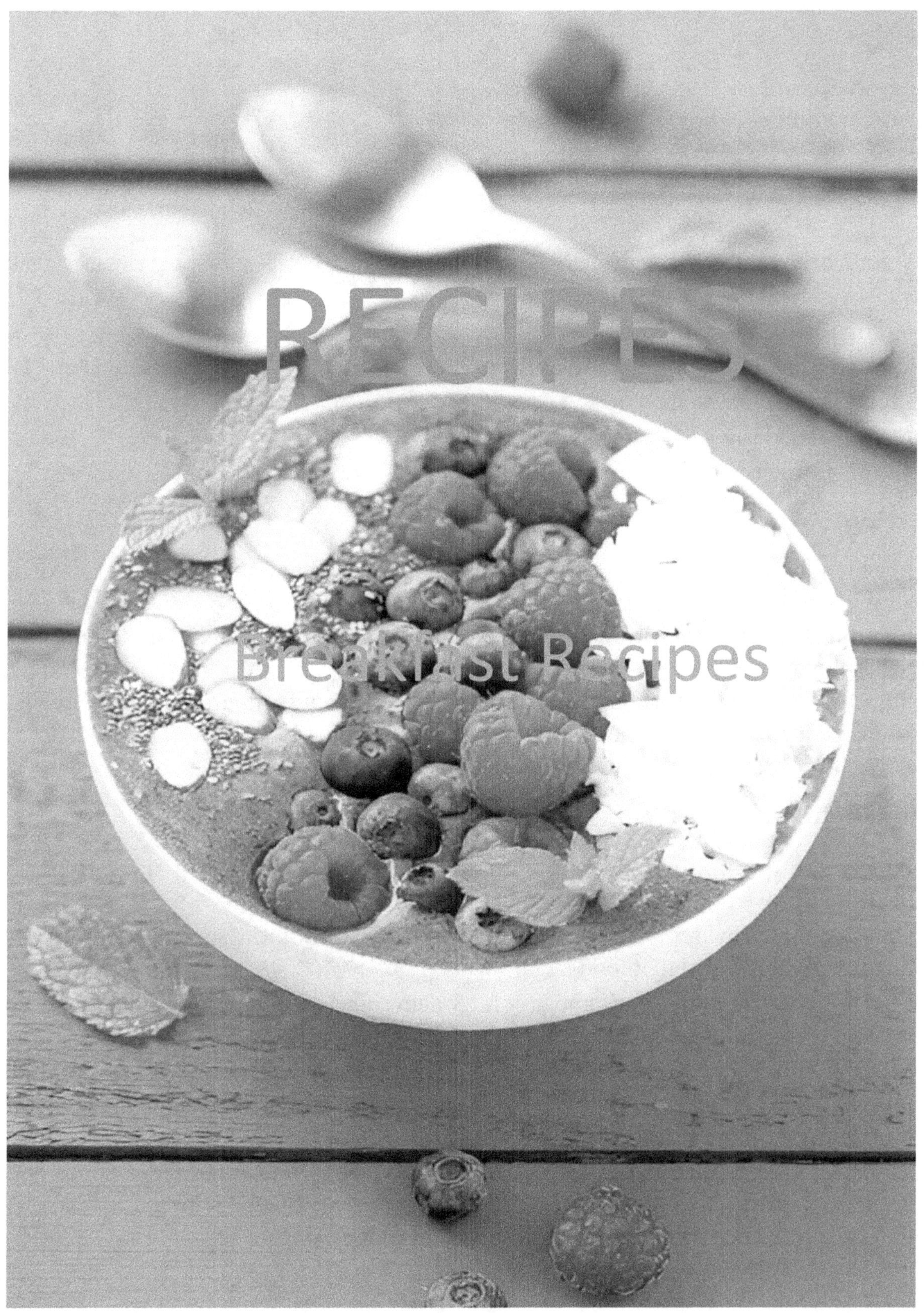
RECIPES
Breakfast Recipes

Berry Blast Smoothie Bowl

Recipe:

Prep Time: 5 minutes
Cook Time: 0 minutes
Number of Servings: 1

Ingredients:

- 1 cup frozen mixed berries (such as strawberries, blueberries, raspberries)
- ½ frozen banana, sliced
- ½ cup plain Greek yogurt
- ¼ cup almond milk (or any milk of your choice)
- 1 tablespoon chia seeds
- 1 tablespoon honey or maple syrup (optional)
- Toppings: sliced fresh fruit, granola, nuts, seeds, shredded coconut

Instructions:

1. In a blender, combine the frozen mixed berries, frozen banana slices, Greek yogurt, almond milk, chia seeds, and honey or maple syrup (if using).
2. Blend on high speed until smooth and creamy, adding more almond milk if needed to reach your desired consistency.
3. Pour the smoothie into a bowl and top with sliced fresh fruit, granola, nuts, seeds, and shredded coconut as desired.
4. Serve immediately and enjoy!

Health Benefits:

- Berries are rich in antioxidants, vitamins, and fiber, which help support heart health, improve digestion, and regulate blood sugar levels.
- Greek yogurt provides a good source of protein and probiotics, which promote gut health and help regulate blood sugar levels.
- Chia seeds are high in fiber, omega-3 fatty acids, and protein, which help promote satiety, regulate blood sugar levels, and support heart health.
- Almond milk is low in calories and carbohydrates, making it a suitable option for individuals with diabetes. It is also fortified with calcium and vitamin D, which are important for bone health.
- Toppings such as sliced fresh fruit, granola, nuts, seeds, and shredded coconut add additional nutrients, fiber, and texture to the smoothie bowl, making it a delicious and nutritious breakfast option for individuals with diabetes.

Turkey and Veggie Breakfast Burritos

Recipe:

Prep Time: 15 minutes
Cook Time: 15 minutes
Number of Servings: 4

Ingredients:

- 4 large whole wheat or low-carb tortillas
- 1 tablespoon olive oil
- 1 small onion, diced
- 1 bell pepper (any color), diced
- 1 cup sliced mushrooms
- 1 cup cooked turkey sausage or ground turkey
- 4 large eggs, beaten
- ½ cup shredded cheddar cheese
- Salt and pepper, to taste
- Salsa and Greek yogurt (optional, for serving)

Instructions:

1. Heat olive oil in a large skillet over medium heat. Add diced onion, bell pepper, and sliced mushrooms, and cook until softened, about 5 minutes.
2. Add cooked turkey sausage or ground turkey to the skillet, and cook until heated through, about 3-4 minutes.
3. Push the vegetables and turkey mixture to one side of the skillet, and pour beaten eggs into the empty side. Cook, stirring occasionally, until the eggs are scrambled and cooked through.
4. Warm the tortillas in the microwave or on a skillet for a few seconds until soft and pliable.
5. Divide the scrambled egg mixture evenly among the tortillas, and sprinkle with shredded cheddar cheese.
6. Roll up the tortillas into burritos, folding in the sides as you roll.
7. Optional: Heat a clean skillet over medium heat and place the burritos seam side down. Cook for 2-3 minutes on each side until lightly browned and crispy.
8. Serve the breakfast burritos with salsa and Greek yogurt on the side, if desired.

Health Benefits:

- Whole wheat tortillas provide fiber and complex carbohydrates, which help regulate blood sugar levels and promote satiety.

- Turkey sausage or ground turkey is a lean protein source that helps stabilize blood sugar levels and promote muscle repair and growth.
- Vegetables like onions, bell peppers, and mushrooms are low in calories and carbohydrates, high in fiber, vitamins, and minerals, and help support overall health and blood sugar control.
- Eggs are a good source of high-quality protein and essential nutrients, making them a nutritious addition to the diet of individuals with diabetes. Protein helps regulate blood sugar levels and promote satiety.
- Greek yogurt is a good source of protein and probiotics, which promote gut health and help regulate blood sugar levels. It is also lower in carbohydrates compared to regular yogurt, making it a suitable option for individuals with diabetes.

These Turkey and Veggie Breakfast Burritos are not only delicious and satisfying but also provide a balanced combination of protein, carbohydrates, and fiber, making them a nutritious breakfast option for individuals with diabetes.

Overnight Chia Seed Pudding with Almond Milk

Recipe:

Prep Time: 5 minutes
Cook Time: 0 minutes (overnight refrigeration required)
Number of Servings: 2

Ingredients:

- ¼ cup chia seeds
- 1 cup unsweetened almond milk (or any milk of your choice)
- 1 tablespoon honey or maple syrup (optional)
- ½ teaspoon vanilla extract
- Fresh fruit, nuts, and seeds for topping (optional)

Instructions:

1. In a mixing bowl, combine chia seeds, almond milk, honey or maple syrup (if using), and vanilla extract. Stir well to combine.
2. Cover the bowl and refrigerate overnight or for at least 4 hours to allow the chia seeds to absorb the liquid and thicken into a pudding-like consistency.
3. Stir the chia seed pudding before serving to ensure an even texture.
4. Divide the pudding into serving bowls and top with fresh fruit, nuts, and seeds as desired.
5. Serve chilled and enjoy!

Health Benefits:

- Chia seeds are rich in fiber, omega-3 fatty acids, protein, vitamins, and minerals, making them an excellent addition to the diet of individuals with diabetes. Fiber helps regulate blood sugar levels and promote satiety, while omega-3 fatty acids support heart health.
- Unsweetened almond milk is low in calories and carbohydrates, making it a suitable option for individuals with diabetes. It is also fortified with calcium and vitamin D, which are important for bone health.
- Honey or maple syrup (if using) adds natural sweetness to the chia seed pudding without causing rapid spikes in blood sugar levels. However, individuals with diabetes should use sweeteners in moderation and adjust according to their personal preferences and blood sugar control.

This Overnight Chia Seed Pudding with Almond Milk is a convenient and nutritious breakfast or snack option for individuals with diabetes. It can be prepared in advance and customized with a variety of toppings to suit individual tastes and preferences while providing essential nutrients and supporting blood sugar control.

Veggie and Cheese Breakfast Muffins

Recipe:

Prep Time: 15 minutes
Cook Time: 25 minutes
Number of Servings: 12 muffins

Ingredients:

- 1 cup whole wheat flour
- 1 teaspoon baking powder
- ½ teaspoon baking soda
- ¼ teaspoon salt
- 4 large eggs
- ½ cup unsweetened almond milk (or any milk of your choice)
- ¼ cup olive oil
- 1 cup chopped vegetables (such as spinach, bell peppers, onions, mushrooms)
- ½ cup shredded cheddar cheese
- Salt and pepper, to taste

Instructions:

1. Preheat the oven to 350°F (175°C). Grease a 12-cup muffin tin or line with paper liners.
2. In a large mixing bowl, whisk together the whole wheat flour, baking powder, baking soda, and salt.
3. In a separate bowl, beat the eggs, then stir in the almond milk and olive oil until well combined.
4. Pour the wet ingredients into the dry ingredients and stir until just combined. Be careful not to overmix.
5. Fold in the chopped vegetables and shredded cheddar cheese until evenly distributed throughout the batter. Season with salt and pepper to taste.
6. Divide the batter evenly among the muffin cups, filling each about 2/3 full.
7. Bake in the preheated oven for 20-25 minutes, or until the muffins are golden brown and a toothpick inserted into the center comes out clean.
8. Remove from the oven and let cool in the muffin tin for a few minutes before transferring to a wire rack to cool completely.
9. Serve warm or at room temperature, and enjoy!

Health Benefits:

- Whole wheat flour provides fiber, vitamins, and minerals compared to refined flour, helping regulate blood sugar levels and promote overall health.

- Eggs are a good source of high-quality protein and essential nutrients, making them a nutritious addition to the diet of individuals with diabetes. Protein helps regulate blood sugar levels and promote satiety.
- Unsweetened almond milk is low in calories and carbohydrates, making it a suitable option for individuals with diabetes. It is also fortified with calcium and vitamin D, which are important for bone health.
- Vegetables such as spinach, bell peppers, onions, and mushrooms are low in calories and carbohydrates, high in fiber, vitamins, and minerals, and help support overall health and blood sugar control.
- Shredded cheddar cheese adds flavor and protein to the muffins, helping stabilize blood sugar levels and promote satiety.

These Veggie and Cheese Breakfast Muffins are a delicious and nutritious option for breakfast or snack time. Packed with vegetables, protein, and whole grains, they provide essential nutrients while supporting blood sugar control and overall health for individuals with diabetes.

Spinach and Feta Omelette

Recipe:

Prep Time: 10 minutes
Cook Time: 5 minutes
Number of Servings: 1

Ingredients:

- 2 large eggs
- 1 tablespoon water or milk
- 1 cup fresh spinach leaves, chopped
- ¼ cup crumbled feta cheese
- Salt and pepper, to taste
- Cooking spray or olive oil

Instructions:

1. In a small mixing bowl, whisk together the eggs and water or milk until well combined. Season with salt and pepper to taste.
2. Heat a non-stick skillet over medium heat and spray with cooking spray or add a drizzle of olive oil.
3. Add the chopped spinach to the skillet and cook until wilted, about 1-2 minutes.
4. Pour the beaten eggs into the skillet, swirling to evenly distribute the mixture.
5. Cook the eggs for 2-3 minutes, or until the edges start to set.
6. Sprinkle the crumbled feta cheese over one half of the omelette.
7. Using a spatula, carefully fold the other half of the omelette over the cheese to create a half-moon shape.
8. Cook for another 1-2 minutes, or until the eggs are fully cooked and the cheese is melted.
9. Slide the omelette onto a plate, and serve hot.

Health Benefits:

- Eggs are a nutritious source of protein, vitamins, and minerals, making them an excellent choice for individuals with diabetes. Protein helps regulate blood sugar levels and promote satiety, while vitamins and minerals support overall health.
- Spinach is low in calories and carbohydrates, high in fiber, vitamins, and minerals, and helps support blood sugar control and overall health. It is also rich in antioxidants, which help protect against oxidative stress and inflammation.
- Feta cheese adds flavor and protein to the omelette, helping stabilize blood sugar levels and promote satiety. It is lower in calories and fat compared to some other cheeses, making it a suitable option for individuals with diabetes.

This Spinach and Feta Omelette is a quick, easy, and nutritious breakfast option for individuals with diabetes. Packed with protein, fiber, and essential nutrients, it provides a satisfying and delicious way to start the day while supporting blood sugar control and overall health.

Peanut Butter Banana Toast

Recipe:

Prep Time: 5 minutes
Cook Time: 5 minutes
Number of Servings: 1

Ingredients:

- 1 slice whole wheat bread (or bread of your choice)
- 1 tablespoon natural peanut butter
- ½ ripe banana, sliced
- Drizzle of honey or maple syrup (optional)
- Pinch of cinnamon (optional)

Instructions:

1. Toast the slice of bread until golden brown and crispy.
2. Spread the natural peanut butter evenly over the toasted bread.
3. Arrange the sliced banana on top of the peanut butter.
4. Drizzle with honey or maple syrup for added sweetness, if desired.
5. Sprinkle with a pinch of cinnamon for extra flavor, if desired.
6. Serve immediately and enjoy!

Health Benefits:

- Whole wheat bread provides fiber and complex carbohydrates, which help regulate blood sugar levels and promote satiety. Choosing whole wheat bread over refined bread ensures you get more nutrients and fiber.
- Natural peanut butter is a good source of healthy fats, protein, and fiber. It helps stabilize blood sugar levels and promotes satiety. Look for peanut butter without added sugars or hydrogenated oils for a healthier option.
- Bananas are a nutritious fruit that provides natural sweetness and essential nutrients like potassium, vitamin C, and vitamin B6. They are low in calories and carbohydrates, making them a suitable option for individuals with diabetes.
- Honey or maple syrup (if using) adds natural sweetness to the toast without causing rapid spikes in blood sugar levels. However, individuals with diabetes should use sweeteners in moderation and adjust according to their personal preferences and blood sugar control.

This Peanut Butter Banana Toast is a simple yet delicious breakfast or snack option for individuals with diabetes. Packed with fiber, healthy fats, and essential nutrients, it provides a satisfying and nutritious way to start the day while supporting blood sugar control and overall health.

Greek Yogurt Pancakes

Recipe:

Prep Time: 10 minutes
Cook Time: 10 minutes
Number of Servings: 4 (makes about 8 pancakes)

Ingredients:

- 1 cup all-purpose flour
- 1 teaspoon baking powder
- ¼ teaspoon baking soda
- ¼ teaspoon salt
- 1 cup plain Greek yogurt
- 2 large eggs
- 1 tablespoon honey or maple syrup (optional)
- 1 teaspoon vanilla extract
- Cooking spray or butter, for greasing the skillet
- Fresh fruit, for serving (optional)
- Maple syrup or honey, for drizzling (optional)

Instructions:

1. In a large mixing bowl, whisk together the all-purpose flour, baking powder, baking soda, and salt.
2. In a separate bowl, combine the plain Greek yogurt, eggs, honey or maple syrup (if using), and vanilla extract. Whisk until smooth and well combined.
3. Pour the wet ingredients into the dry ingredients and stir until just combined. Be careful not to overmix; the batter should be slightly lumpy.
4. Heat a non-stick skillet or griddle over medium heat and lightly grease with cooking spray or butter.
5. Pour about ¼ cup of batter onto the skillet for each pancake. Cook until bubbles form on the surface of the pancake and the edges begin to set, about 2-3 minutes.
6. Flip the pancakes and cook for an additional 1-2 minutes, or until golden brown and cooked through.
7. Remove the pancakes from the skillet and keep warm. Repeat with the remaining batter, greasing the skillet as needed.
8. Serve the Greek yogurt pancakes warm, topped with fresh fruit and a drizzle of maple syrup or honey, if desired.

Health Benefits:

- Greek yogurt is a good source of protein and probiotics, which promote gut health and help regulate blood sugar levels. It also adds creaminess and moisture to the pancakes without the need for additional fat.
- All-purpose flour is used in moderation to provide structure to the pancakes. However, you can substitute whole wheat flour or a combination of whole wheat and all-purpose flour for added fiber and nutrients.
- Eggs provide protein and essential nutrients, making them a nutritious addition to the pancakes. Protein helps regulate blood sugar levels and promote satiety.
- Honey or maple syrup (if using) adds natural sweetness to the pancakes without causing rapid spikes in blood sugar levels. However, individuals with diabetes should use sweeteners in moderation and adjust according to their personal preferences and blood sugar control.

These Greek Yogurt Pancakes are light, fluffy, and delicious, making them a perfect breakfast or brunch option for individuals with diabetes. Packed with protein, they provide long-lasting energy and help stabilize blood sugar levels while satisfying your pancake cravings. Serve them with fresh fruit and a drizzle of maple syrup or honey for a nutritious and satisfying meal.

Egg and Avocado Breakfast Wrap

Recipe:

Prep Time: 5 minutes
Cook Time: 5 minutes
Number of Servings: 1

Ingredients:

- 1 large whole wheat or low-carb tortilla
- 1 large egg
- ½ ripe avocado, sliced
- 1 tablespoon diced tomatoes
- 1 tablespoon diced red onion
- 1 tablespoon chopped fresh cilantro or parsley
- Salt and pepper, to taste
- Cooking spray or olive oil

Instructions:

1. Heat a non-stick skillet over medium heat and lightly grease with cooking spray or olive oil.
2. Crack the egg into the skillet and cook to your desired doneness (scrambled, fried, or poached).
3. While the egg is cooking, warm the tortilla in a separate skillet or microwave until soft and pliable.
4. Once the egg is cooked, transfer it to the center of the tortilla.
5. Top the egg with sliced avocado, diced tomatoes, diced red onion, and chopped fresh cilantro or parsley.
6. Season with salt and pepper to taste.
7. Fold the sides of the tortilla over the filling to create a wrap.
8. Serve the egg and avocado breakfast wrap immediately, and enjoy!

Health Benefits:

- Whole wheat or low-carb tortilla provides fiber and complex carbohydrates, which help regulate blood sugar levels and promote satiety. Choosing whole wheat or low-carb tortillas over refined tortillas ensures you get more nutrients and fiber.
- Eggs are a good source of high-quality protein and essential nutrients, making them a nutritious addition to the diet of individuals with diabetes. Protein helps regulate blood sugar levels and promote satiety.

- Avocado is rich in heart-healthy monounsaturated fats, fiber, vitamins, and minerals. It helps stabilize blood sugar levels, promote satiety, and support overall heart health.
- Tomatoes and red onions add flavor, texture, and nutrients to the breakfast wrap. They are low in calories and carbohydrates, high in fiber, vitamins, and antioxidants, and help support overall health and blood sugar control.
- Fresh cilantro or parsley adds a burst of flavor and freshness to the breakfast wrap. It is low in calories and carbohydrates, high in antioxidants, vitamins, and minerals, and helps support overall health and blood sugar control.

This Egg and Avocado Breakfast Wrap is a quick, easy, and nutritious meal option for individuals with diabetes. Packed with protein, healthy fats, fiber, and essential nutrients, it provides a satisfying and delicious way to start the day while supporting blood sugar control and overall health.

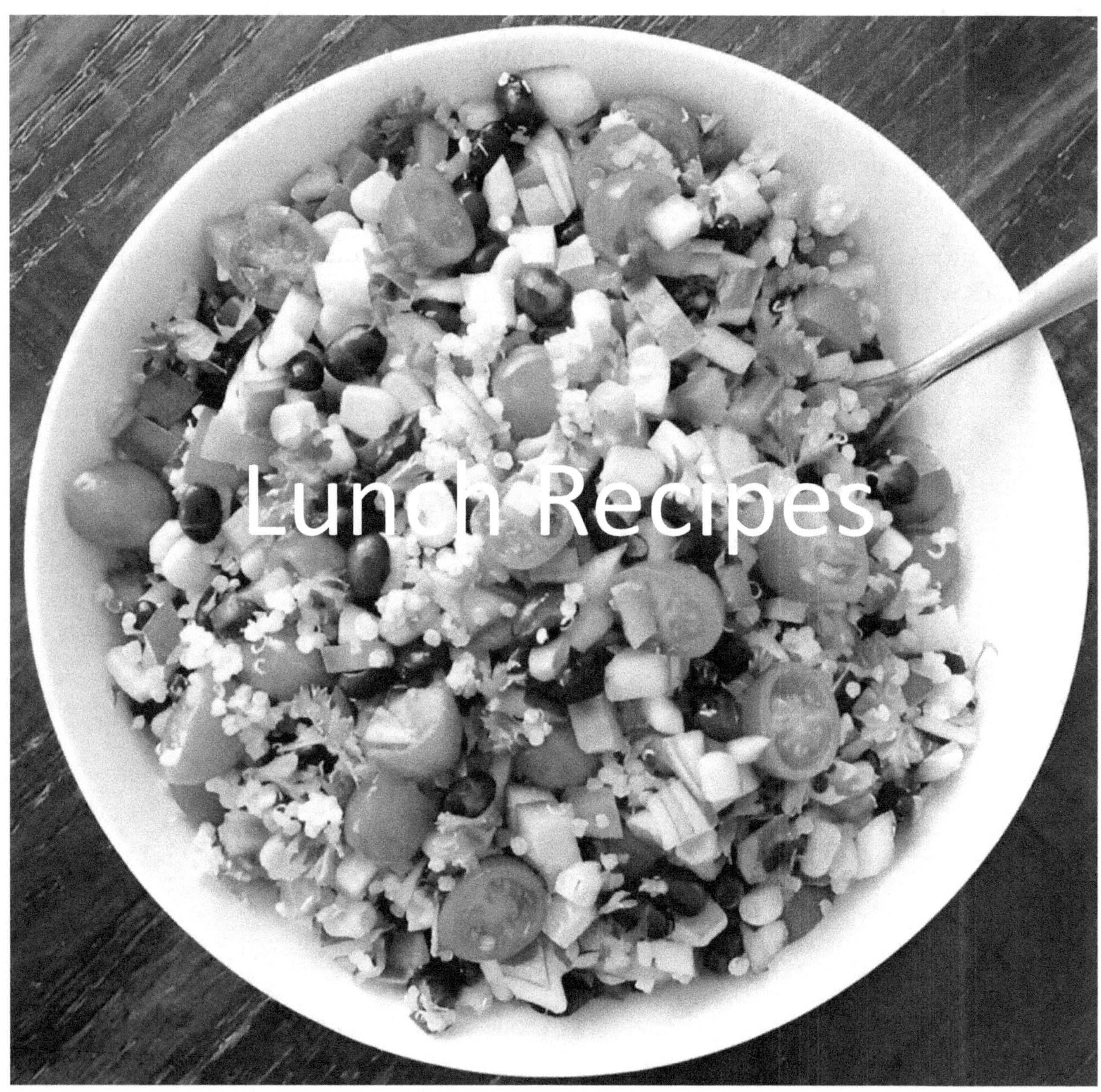
Lunch Recipes

Quinoa and Black Bean Salad

Recipes

Prep Time: 15 minutes
Cook Time: 15 minutes
Number of Servings: 4

Ingredients:

- 1 cup quinoa, rinsed
- 2 cups water or vegetable broth
- 1 can (15 ounces) black beans, drained and rinsed
- 1 cup cherry tomatoes, halved
- 1 red bell pepper, diced
- ¼ cup chopped red onion
- ¼ cup chopped fresh cilantro
- 1 jalapeño, seeded and diced (optional for added spice)
- 2 tablespoons extra-virgin olive oil
- 2 tablespoons lime juice
- 1 teaspoon ground cumin
- ½ teaspoon chili powder
- Salt and pepper, to taste
- Avocado slices, for garnish (optional)

Instructions:

1. In a medium saucepan, combine the quinoa and water or vegetable broth. Bring to a boil over medium-high heat, then reduce the heat to low, cover, and simmer for 12-15 minutes, or until the quinoa is tender and the liquid is absorbed. Remove from heat and let it cool slightly.
2. In a large mixing bowl, combine the cooked quinoa, black beans, cherry tomatoes, red bell pepper, red onion, chopped cilantro, and diced jalapeño (if using). Toss gently to combine.
3. In a small mixing bowl, whisk together the extra-virgin olive oil, lime juice, ground cumin, chili powder, salt, and pepper to create the dressing.
4. Pour the dressing over the quinoa and black bean salad and toss until well coated.
5. If desired, garnish with avocado slices before serving.
6. Serve the salad immediately or refrigerate for at least 30 minutes to allow the flavors to meld.
7. Enjoy as a main dish or side dish!

Health Benefits:

- Quinoa is a gluten-free whole grain that is high in protein, fiber, vitamins, and minerals. It helps regulate blood sugar levels, promote satiety, and support overall health.
- Black beans are a good source of plant-based protein, fiber, vitamins, and minerals. They help stabilize blood sugar levels, promote satiety, and support digestive health.
- Cherry tomatoes, red bell pepper, red onion, and cilantro add freshness, flavor, and nutrients to the salad. They are low in calories and carbohydrates, high in fiber, vitamins, and antioxidants, and help support overall health and blood sugar control.
- Jalapeño (if using) adds a spicy kick to the salad. It contains capsaicin, which has been shown to have anti-inflammatory and metabolism-boosting properties.
- Extra-virgin olive oil provides healthy fats and antioxidants, which help reduce inflammation and promote heart health. It also adds richness and flavor to the salad dressing.

This Quinoa and Black Bean Salad is a nutritious and flavorful meal option for individuals with diabetes. Packed with protein, fiber, vitamins, and minerals, it provides a balanced combination of nutrients while supporting blood sugar control and overall health. Serve it as a main dish or side dish for a satisfying and delicious meal!

Turkey and Avocado Wrap

Recipe:

Prep Time: 10 minutes
Cook Time: 0 minutes
Number of Servings: 1

Ingredients:

- 1 large whole wheat or low-carb tortilla
- 2-3 slices of cooked turkey breast
- ¼ ripe avocado, sliced
- ¼ cup baby spinach leaves
- 1 tablespoon hummus or Greek yogurt spread
- 1 tablespoon diced tomatoes
- Salt and pepper, to taste

Instructions:

1. Lay the tortilla flat on a clean surface.
2. Spread the hummus or Greek yogurt spread evenly over the tortilla, leaving about 1-inch border around the edges.
3. Layer the cooked turkey breast slices, sliced avocado, baby spinach leaves, and diced tomatoes on top of the spread.
4. Season with salt and pepper to taste.
5. Starting from one side, tightly roll the tortilla into a wrap, tucking in the fillings as you go.
6. Slice the wrap in half diagonally, if desired, and serve immediately.

Health Benefits:

- Whole wheat or low-carb tortilla provides fiber and complex carbohydrates, which help regulate blood sugar levels and promote satiety.
- Cooked turkey breast is a lean protein source that helps stabilize blood sugar levels and promote muscle repair and growth.
- Avocado is rich in heart-healthy monounsaturated fats, fiber, vitamins, and minerals. It helps stabilize blood sugar levels, promote satiety, and support overall heart health.
- Baby spinach leaves are low in calories and carbohydrates, high in fiber, vitamins, and minerals, and help support overall health and blood sugar control.
- Hummus or Greek yogurt spread adds flavor and creaminess to the wrap without the need for additional fat or calories.

This Turkey and Avocado Wrap is a quick, easy, and nutritious meal option for individuals with diabetes. Packed with protein, healthy fats, fiber, and essential nutrients, it provides a satisfying and delicious way to enjoy a balanced meal while supporting blood sugar control and overall health. Enjoy it for lunch, dinner, or as a portable snack on the go!

Garlic Roasted Broccoli with Lemon

Recipe:

Prep Time: 10 minutes
Cook Time: 20 minutes
Number of Servings: 4

Ingredients:

- 1 pound broccoli florets
- 3 cloves garlic, minced
- 2 tablespoons olive oil
- 1 tablespoon lemon juice
- Zest of 1 lemon
- Salt and pepper, to taste

Instructions:

1. Preheat the oven to 425°F (220°C). Line a baking sheet with parchment paper or aluminum foil.
2. In a large bowl, toss the broccoli florets with minced garlic, olive oil, lemon juice, lemon zest, salt, and pepper until evenly coated.
3. Spread the broccoli mixture in a single layer on the prepared baking sheet.
4. Roast in the preheated oven for 15-20 minutes, or until the broccoli is tender and lightly browned, stirring halfway through cooking.
5. Remove from the oven and transfer the roasted broccoli to a serving dish.
6. Serve hot as a side dish or garnish with additional lemon zest before serving.

Health Benefits:

This recipe is rich in fiber, vitamins, and minerals from the broccoli. Garlic provides anti-inflammatory and immune-boosting properties. Olive oil adds heart-healthy monounsaturated fats, and lemon juice adds vitamin C and brightness to the dish. The combination of ingredients supports overall health and may help regulate blood sugar levels.

Greek Yogurt Parfait with Nuts and Berries

Recipe:

Prep Time: 5 minutes
Cook Time: 0 minutes
Number of Servings: 1

Ingredients:

- ½ cup plain Greek yogurt
- ¼ cup mixed nuts (such as almonds, walnuts, or pecans), chopped
- ¼ cup mixed berries (such as strawberries, blueberries, or raspberries)
- 1 tablespoon honey or maple syrup (optional)

Instructions:

1. In a serving glass or bowl, layer the plain Greek yogurt, mixed nuts, and mixed berries.
2. Drizzle with honey or maple syrup if desired.
3. Repeat the layers until the glass or bowl is filled.
4. Serve immediately as a delicious and nutritious breakfast or snack.

Health Benefits:

This recipe is high in protein from the Greek yogurt and nuts, which helps regulate blood sugar levels and promotes satiety. The nuts provide healthy fats, fiber, and essential nutrients, contributing to heart health and overall well-being. Berries are low in calories and carbohydrates, high in fiber, vitamins, and antioxidants, and help support overall health and blood sugar control. The combination of ingredients offers a balance of nutrients and flavors for a satisfying and delicious parfait.

Chicken Caesar Salad

Recipe:

Prep Time: 15 minutes
Cook Time: 15 minutes
Number of Servings: 4

Ingredients:

- 2 boneless, skinless chicken breasts
- 1 tablespoon olive oil
- Salt and pepper, to taste
- 1 head romaine lettuce, chopped
- ½ cup cherry tomatoes, halved
- ¼ cup grated Parmesan cheese
- ¼ cup Caesar salad dressing (homemade or store-bought)
- ¼ cup croutons (optional)

Instructions:

1. Preheat the oven to 375°F (190°C). Line a baking sheet with parchment paper.
2. Brush the chicken breasts with olive oil and season with salt and pepper.
3. Place the chicken breasts on the prepared baking sheet and bake in the preheated oven for 15-20 minutes, or until cooked through and no longer pink in the center. Remove from the oven and let cool slightly.
4. Slice the cooked chicken breasts into thin strips.
5. In a large mixing bowl, combine the chopped romaine lettuce, cherry tomatoes, grated Parmesan cheese, and sliced chicken breasts.
6. Drizzle the Caesar salad dressing over the salad and toss until well coated.
7. Optional: Add croutons for extra crunch and flavor.
8. Serve the Chicken Caesar Salad immediately as a delicious and satisfying meal.

Health Benefits:

This recipe is high in protein from the chicken, which helps regulate blood sugar levels and promotes satiety. Romaine lettuce provides fiber, vitamins, and minerals, contributing to overall health and blood sugar control. Cherry tomatoes add freshness, flavor, and antioxidants to the salad. Parmesan cheese adds calcium and flavor. The Caesar salad dressing adds creaminess and flavor to the salad. This Chicken Caesar Salad is a balanced and nutritious meal option for individuals with diabetes.

Tuna Salad Lettuce Wraps

Recipe:

Prep Time: 10 minutes
Cook Time: 0 minutes
Number of Servings: 2

Ingredients:

- 1 can (5 ounces) tuna, drained
- 2 tablespoons mayonnaise or Greek yogurt
- 1 tablespoon Dijon mustard
- ¼ cup diced celery
- ¼ cup diced red onion
- ¼ cup diced pickles
- Salt and pepper, to taste
- 4 large lettuce leaves (such as romaine or butter lettuce)

Instructions:

1. In a mixing bowl, combine the drained tuna, mayonnaise or Greek yogurt, Dijon mustard, diced celery, diced red onion, and diced pickles. Mix well to combine.
2. Season with salt and pepper to taste.
3. Place a spoonful of the tuna salad mixture onto each lettuce leaf.
4. Roll up the lettuce leaves to create lettuce wraps.
5. Serve immediately as a delicious and low-carb meal or snack.

Health Benefits:

This recipe is high in protein from the tuna, which helps regulate blood sugar levels and promotes satiety. Tuna is also a good source of omega-3 fatty acids, which have been shown to have heart-healthy benefits. The addition of celery, red onion, and pickles adds fiber, vitamins, and minerals to the salad, contributing to overall health and blood sugar control. Using Greek yogurt instead of mayonnaise reduces the calorie and fat content of the salad while adding probiotics and protein. Serving the tuna salad in lettuce wraps instead of bread or tortillas reduces the carbohydrate content of the meal and adds extra fiber and nutrients. Overall, these Tuna Salad Lettuce Wraps are a nutritious and satisfying option for individuals with diabetes.

Caprese Salad with Balsamic Glaze

Recipe :

Prep Time: 10 minutes
Cook Time: 0 minutes
Number of Servings: 4

Ingredients:

- 2 large tomatoes, sliced
- 1 ball fresh mozzarella cheese, sliced
- ¼ cup fresh basil leaves
- 2 tablespoons balsamic glaze
- Salt and pepper, to taste

Instructions:

1. Arrange the tomato slices and mozzarella slices alternately on a serving platter.
2. Tuck fresh basil leaves between the tomato and mozzarella slices.
3. Drizzle balsamic glaze over the tomato and mozzarella slices.
4. Season with salt and pepper to taste.
5. Serve immediately as a refreshing and flavorful appetizer or side dish.

Health Benefits:

This recipe is rich in vitamins, minerals, and antioxidants from the tomatoes, fresh mozzarella cheese, and basil leaves. Tomatoes are a good source of vitamin C, potassium, and antioxidants, which help support overall health and blood sugar control. Fresh mozzarella cheese adds protein and calcium to the salad, promoting satiety and bone health. Basil leaves add flavor and essential nutrients to the salad, including vitamin K and antioxidants. The balsamic glaze adds sweetness and acidity to the salad without adding extra sugar or calories. Overall, this Caprese Salad with Balsamic Glaze is a delicious and nutritious option for individuals with diabetes.

Lentil Vegetable Soup

Recipe:

Prep Time: 15 minutes
Cook Time: 45 minutes
Number of Servings: 6

Ingredients:

- 1 cup dried lentils, rinsed
- 1 tablespoon olive oil
- 1 onion, diced
- 2 carrots, diced
- 2 celery stalks, diced
- 3 cloves garlic, minced
- 1 can (14.5 ounces) diced tomatoes
- 6 cups vegetable broth
- 1 teaspoon dried thyme
- 1 teaspoon dried oregano
- 1 bay leaf
- Salt and pepper, to taste
- 2 cups chopped spinach or kale
- Juice of 1 lemon (optional)
- Fresh parsley, for garnish (optional)

Instructions:

1. In a large pot, heat olive oil over medium heat. Add diced onion, carrots, and celery, and cook until softened, about 5 minutes.
2. Add minced garlic and cook for an additional 1-2 minutes, until fragrant.
3. Stir in dried lentils, diced tomatoes, vegetable broth, dried thyme, dried oregano, bay leaf, salt, and pepper.
4. Bring the soup to a boil, then reduce heat to low and simmer, covered, for 30-40 minutes, or until the lentils are tender.
5. Stir in chopped spinach or kale and simmer for an additional 5 minutes, until wilted.
6. Remove the bay leaf from the soup and discard.
7. If desired, stir in lemon juice for a bright, citrusy flavor.
8. Ladle the soup into bowls and garnish with fresh parsley, if using.
9. Serve hot and enjoy!

Health Benefits: This Lentil Vegetable Soup is high in fiber and plant-based protein from the lentils, which help regulate blood sugar levels and promote satiety. It is also packed with vitamins, minerals, and antioxidants from the vegetables, including carrots, celery, tomatoes, spinach, and kale, which support overall health and blood sugar control. Olive oil adds heart-healthy monounsaturated fats, and lemon juice adds vitamin C and brightness to the soup. The combination of ingredients offers a delicious and nutritious meal option for individuals with diabetes.

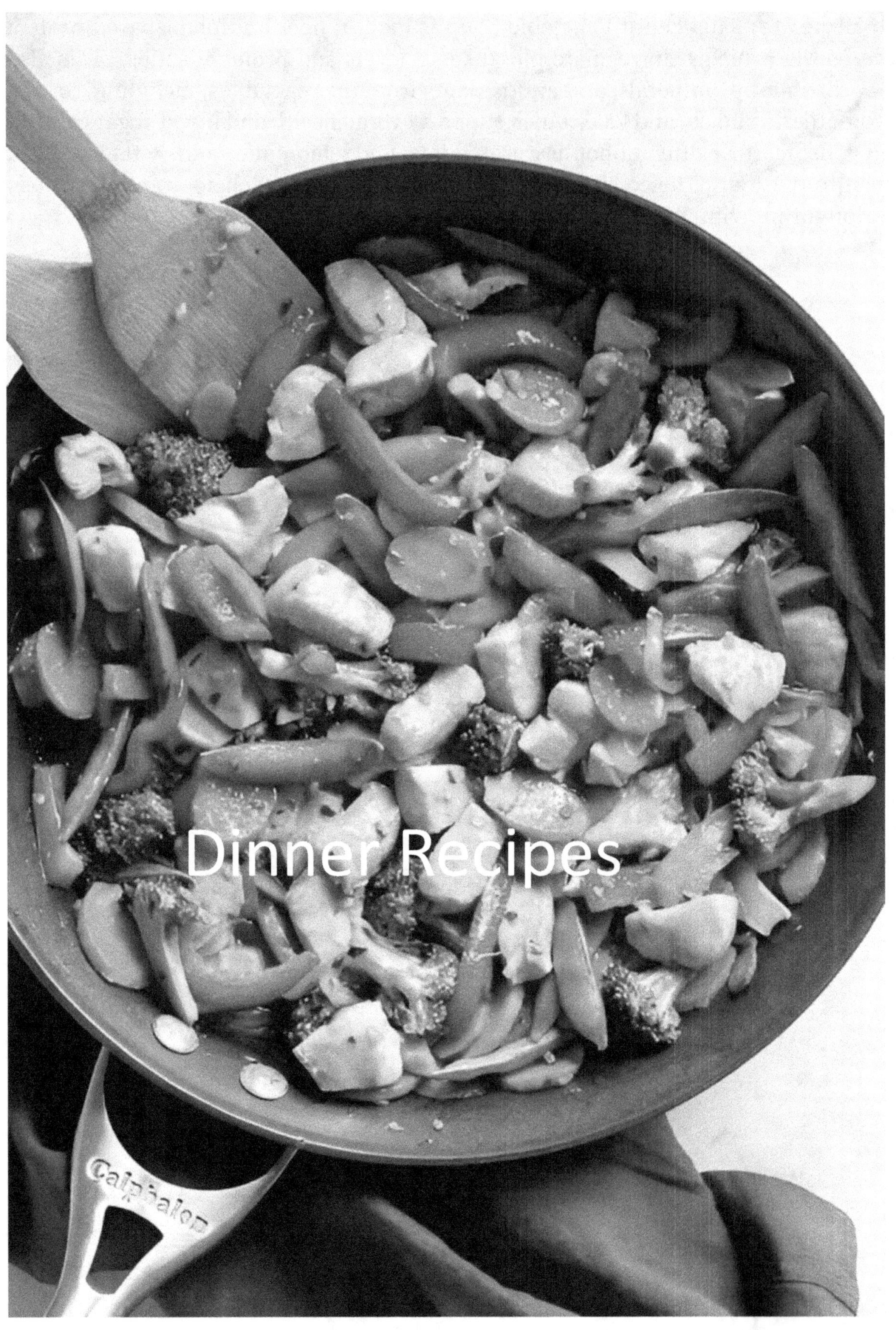
Dinner Recipes

Salmon with Dill Sauce

Recipe:

Prep Time: 10 minutes
Cook Time: 15 minutes
Number of Servings: 4

Ingredients:

- 4 salmon fillets (about 6 ounces each)
- Salt and pepper, to taste
- 2 tablespoons olive oil
- ¼ cup plain Greek yogurt
- 2 tablespoons chopped fresh dill
- 1 tablespoon lemon juice
- 1 teaspoon Dijon mustard
- 1 clove garlic, minced

Instructions:

1. Preheat the oven to 400°F (200°C). Line a baking sheet with parchment paper.
2. Place the salmon fillets on the prepared baking sheet. Season with salt and pepper to taste.
3. Drizzle olive oil over the salmon fillets.
4. Bake in the preheated oven for 12-15 minutes, or until the salmon is cooked through and flakes easily with a fork.
5. While the salmon is baking, prepare the dill sauce. In a small mixing bowl, combine the plain Greek yogurt, chopped fresh dill, lemon juice, Dijon mustard, and minced garlic. Mix well to combine.
6. Remove the salmon from the oven and transfer to serving plates.
7. Spoon the dill sauce over the cooked salmon fillets.
8. Serve immediately with your favorite side dishes.

Health Benefits:-

This recipe is rich in omega-3 fatty acids from the salmon, which have been shown to have heart-healthy benefits and may help reduce inflammation. Salmon is also a good source of high-quality protein, which helps regulate blood sugar levels and promotes satiety. The dill sauce adds flavor and creaminess to the dish without the need for additional fat or calories. Greek yogurt provides probiotics and protein, contributing to gut health and satiety. Overall, this Salmon with Dill Sauce is a delicious and nutritious option for individuals with diabetes.

Chicken and Vegetable Stir-Fry

Recipe:

Prep Time: 15 minutes
Cook Time: 15 minutes
Number of Servings: 4

Ingredients:

- 1 pound boneless, skinless chicken breasts, thinly sliced
- 2 tablespoons soy sauce (or tamari for gluten-free option)
- 1 tablespoon rice vinegar
- 1 tablespoon cornstarch
- 2 tablespoons olive oil, divided
- 2 cloves garlic, minced
- 1 tablespoon grated ginger
- 1 red bell pepper, sliced
- 1 yellow bell pepper, sliced
- 1 cup snow peas, trimmed
- 1 cup broccoli florets
- 1 medium carrot, sliced
- Cooked rice or quinoa, for serving

Instructions:

1. In a small bowl, whisk together the soy sauce, rice vinegar, and cornstarch. Set aside.
2. Heat 1 tablespoon of olive oil in a large skillet or wok over medium-high heat.
3. Add the sliced chicken to the skillet and cook until browned and cooked through, about 5-7 minutes. Remove the chicken from the skillet and set aside.
4. In the same skillet, heat the remaining tablespoon of olive oil.
5. Add the minced garlic and grated ginger to the skillet and cook for 1 minute, until fragrant.
6. Add the sliced bell peppers, snow peas, broccoli florets, and sliced carrot to the skillet. Stir-fry for 5-7 minutes, until the vegetables are tender-crisp.
7. Return the cooked chicken to the skillet.
8. Pour the soy sauce mixture over the chicken and vegetables. Stir well to coat everything evenly.
9. Cook for an additional 2-3 minutes, until the sauce has thickened slightly.
10. Serve the chicken and vegetable stir-fry hot over cooked rice or quinoa.

Health Benefits:-

This Chicken and Vegetable Stir-Fry is a balanced and nutritious meal option for individuals with diabetes. It is packed with lean protein from the chicken and a variety of colorful vegetables, providing essential vitamins, minerals, and antioxidants. The use of olive oil as the cooking fat adds heart-healthy monounsaturated fats, while the soy sauce mixture adds flavor without adding extra sodium or sugar. Serving the stir-fry over cooked rice or quinoa provides complex carbohydrates and fiber, promoting satiety and helping to regulate blood sugar levels. Overall, this stir-fry is a delicious and satisfying option for a healthy meal.

Stuffed Bell Peppers with Quinoa and Ground Turkey

Recipe:

Prep Time: 20 minutes
Cook Time: 40 minutes
Number of Servings: 4

Ingredients:

- 4 large bell peppers (any color)
- 1 cup quinoa, rinsed
- 2 cups water or vegetable broth
- 1 tablespoon olive oil
- 1 small onion, diced
- 2 cloves garlic, minced
- 1 pound ground turkey
- 1 can (14.5 ounces) diced tomatoes, drained
- 1 teaspoon dried oregano
- 1 teaspoon dried basil
- Salt and pepper, to taste
- ½ cup shredded mozzarella cheese (optional)

Instructions:

1. Preheat the oven to 375°F (190°C). Grease a baking dish large enough to hold the bell peppers.
2. Cut the tops off the bell peppers and remove the seeds and membranes. Place the bell peppers in the prepared baking dish.
3. In a medium saucepan, combine the quinoa and water or vegetable broth. Bring to a boil, then reduce the heat to low, cover, and simmer for 15 minutes, or until the quinoa is cooked and the liquid is absorbed. Remove from heat and set aside.
4. In a large skillet, heat the olive oil over medium heat. Add the diced onion and minced garlic, and cook until softened, about 5 minutes.
5. Add the ground turkey to the skillet and cook until browned and cooked through, breaking it up with a spoon as it cooks.
6. Stir in the diced tomatoes, cooked quinoa, dried oregano, dried basil, salt, and pepper. Cook for an additional 5 minutes, until heated through and well combined.
7. Spoon the turkey and quinoa mixture evenly into the bell peppers, packing it down slightly.
8. If using, sprinkle shredded mozzarella cheese over the tops of the stuffed bell peppers.

9. Cover the baking dish with aluminum foil and bake in the preheated oven for 25-30 minutes, or until the bell peppers are tender.
10. Remove the foil and bake for an additional 5 minutes, or until the cheese is melted and bubbly.
11. Serve the stuffed bell peppers hot, garnished with fresh herbs if desired.

Health Benefits:-

These Stuffed Bell Peppers with Quinoa and Ground Turkey are a nutritious and satisfying meal option for individuals with diabetes. They are packed with lean protein from the ground turkey and fiber-rich quinoa, which help regulate blood sugar levels and promote satiety. Bell peppers are low in calories and carbohydrates, high in fiber, vitamins, and antioxidants, and help support overall health and blood sugar control. This recipe is also versatile and customizable, allowing you to add your favorite herbs, spices, and toppings to suit your taste preferences. Overall, these stuffed bell peppers are a delicious and wholesome option for a balanced meal.

Spaghetti Squash with Turkey Meatballs and Marinara Sauce

Recipe :

Prep Time: 20 minutes
Cook Time: 1 hour
Number of Servings: 4

Ingredients:

- 1 large spaghetti squash
- 1 pound ground turkey
- ¼ cup grated Parmesan cheese
- ¼ cup breadcrumbs (use gluten-free breadcrumbs if needed)
- 1 egg, lightly beaten
- 1 teaspoon dried oregano
- 1 teaspoon dried basil
- ½ teaspoon garlic powder
- Salt and pepper, to taste
- 2 cups marinara sauce (homemade or store-bought)
- Fresh parsley, for garnish (optional)

Instructions:

1. Preheat the oven to 375°F (190°C). Line a baking sheet with parchment paper.
2. Cut the spaghetti squash in half lengthwise and scoop out the seeds.
3. Place the spaghetti squash halves cut-side down on the prepared baking sheet.
4. Bake in the preheated oven for 45-50 minutes, or until the squash is tender and easily pierced with a fork.
5. While the spaghetti squash is baking, prepare the turkey meatballs. In a large mixing bowl, combine the ground turkey, grated Parmesan cheese, breadcrumbs, beaten egg, dried oregano, dried basil, garlic powder, salt, and pepper. Mix well until combined.
6. Shape the turkey mixture into small meatballs, about 1 inch in diameter.
7. Heat a large skillet over medium heat. Add the turkey meatballs to the skillet and cook until browned on all sides and cooked through, about 10-12 minutes.
8. In a separate saucepan, heat the marinara sauce over medium heat until warmed through.
9. Once the spaghetti squash is cooked, use a fork to scrape the flesh into strands.
10. Divide the spaghetti squash strands among serving plates or bowls.
11. Top the spaghetti squash with turkey meatballs and marinara sauce.
12. Garnish with fresh parsley, if desired, and serve hot.

Health Benefits:-

This Spaghetti Squash with Turkey Meatballs and Marinara Sauce is a nutritious and low-carb alternative to traditional pasta dishes. Spaghetti squash is low in calories and carbohydrates, high in fiber, vitamins, and minerals, and helps support blood sugar control and weight management. Turkey meatballs are lean and protein-rich, which helps regulate blood sugar levels and promotes satiety. Using homemade or store-bought marinara sauce without added sugars or preservatives adds flavor and essential nutrients to the dish. Overall, this recipe is a delicious and wholesome option for individuals with diabetes.

Grilled Lemon Herb Chicken

Recipe:

Prep Time: 10 minutes
Cook Time: 15 minutes
Number of Servings: 4

Ingredients:

- 4 boneless, skinless chicken breasts
- 2 tablespoons olive oil
- 2 cloves garlic, minced
- 2 tablespoons chopped fresh herbs (such as rosemary, thyme, and parsley)
- Zest and juice of 1 lemon
- Salt and pepper, to taste

Instructions:

1. In a small bowl, whisk together the olive oil, minced garlic, chopped fresh herbs, lemon zest, lemon juice, salt, and pepper to create the marinade.
2. Place the chicken breasts in a shallow dish or resealable plastic bag.
3. Pour the marinade over the chicken breasts, making sure they are evenly coated. Marinate in the refrigerator for at least 30 minutes, or up to 4 hours, turning occasionally.
4. Preheat the grill to medium-high heat.
5. Remove the chicken breasts from the marinade and discard any excess marinade.
6. Grill the chicken breasts for 6-8 minutes per side, or until cooked through and no longer pink in the center, with an internal temperature of 165°F (74°C).
7. Remove the chicken breasts from the grill and let them rest for a few minutes before serving.
8. Serve the grilled lemon herb chicken hot, garnished with additional fresh herbs if desired.

Health Benefits:-

This Grilled Lemon Herb Chicken is a healthy and flavorful option for individuals with diabetes. Chicken breast is a lean protein source that helps regulate blood sugar levels and promotes satiety. Olive oil provides heart-healthy monounsaturated fats, while fresh herbs add flavor and essential nutrients without adding extra calories or carbohydrates. Lemon juice adds brightness and acidity to the marinade, enhancing the flavor of the chicken. Overall, this recipe is a delicious and nutritious addition to any meal.

Baked Cod with Tomato and Basil

Recipe :

Prep Time: 10 minutes
Cook Time: 20 minutes
Number of Servings: 4

Ingredients:

- 4 cod fillets (about 6 ounces each)
- Salt and pepper, to taste
- 2 tablespoons olive oil
- 2 cloves garlic, minced
- 1 pint cherry tomatoes, halved
- ¼ cup chopped fresh basil leaves
- Zest and juice of 1 lemon

Instructions:

1. Preheat the oven to 400°F (200°C). Line a baking sheet with parchment paper.
2. Season the cod fillets with salt and pepper to taste.
3. Place the cod fillets on the prepared baking sheet.
4. In a small bowl, whisk together the olive oil, minced garlic, cherry tomatoes, chopped fresh basil leaves, lemon zest, and lemon juice.
5. Spoon the tomato and basil mixture over the cod fillets, covering them evenly.
6. Bake in the preheated oven for 15-20 minutes, or until the cod is cooked through and flakes easily with a fork.
7. Remove from the oven and let the cod rest for a few minutes before serving.
8. Serve the baked cod with tomato and basil hot, garnished with additional fresh basil leaves if desired.

Health Benefits:-

This Baked Cod with Tomato and Basil is a light and flavorful dish that's perfect for individuals with diabetes. Cod is a lean protein source that helps regulate blood sugar levels and promotes satiety. Olive oil provides heart-healthy monounsaturated fats, while garlic, cherry tomatoes, and fresh basil add flavor and essential nutrients without adding extra calories or carbohydrates. Lemon zest and juice add brightness and acidity to the dish, enhancing the flavors of the cod and tomatoes. Overall, this recipe is a delicious and nutritious option for a balanced meal.

Vegetable and Chickpea Curry

Recipe:

Prep Time: 15 minutes
Cook Time: 25 minutes
Number of Servings: 4

Ingredients:

- 1 tablespoon olive oil
- 1 onion, diced
- 2 cloves garlic, minced
- 1 tablespoon grated ginger
- 2 tablespoons curry powder
- 1 teaspoon ground turmeric
- 1 teaspoon ground cumin
- 1 teaspoon ground coriander
- ½ teaspoon chili powder (optional, adjust to taste)
- 1 can (14 ounces) chickpeas, drained and rinsed
- 1 can (14.5 ounces) diced tomatoes
- 1 cup vegetable broth
- 1 small head cauliflower, cut into florets
- 2 carrots, sliced
- 1 cup frozen peas
- Salt and pepper, to taste
- Cooked rice or naan, for serving

Instructions:

1. Heat olive oil in a large skillet or pot over medium heat.
2. Add diced onion and cook until softened, about 5 minutes.
3. Add minced garlic and grated ginger, and cook for an additional 1-2 minutes, until fragrant.
4. Stir in curry powder, ground turmeric, ground cumin, ground coriander, and chili powder (if using), and cook for another minute, stirring constantly.
5. Add drained and rinsed chickpeas, diced tomatoes, and vegetable broth to the skillet. Bring to a simmer.
6. Add cauliflower florets and sliced carrots to the skillet. Cover and cook for 10-15 minutes, or until the vegetables are tender.
7. Stir in frozen peas and cook for an additional 2-3 minutes, until heated through.
8. Season with salt and pepper to taste.

9. Serve the vegetable and chickpea curry hot over cooked rice or with naan bread.

Health Benefits:-

This Vegetable and Chickpea Curry is a nutritious and flavorful option for individuals with diabetes. Chickpeas are a good source of protein and fiber, which help regulate blood sugar levels and promote satiety. Cauliflower, carrots, and peas provide vitamins, minerals, and antioxidants, supporting overall health and blood sugar control. Olive oil adds heart-healthy monounsaturated fats, while spices like curry powder, turmeric, cumin, coriander, and chili powder (optional) add flavor and additional health benefits. Serving the curry over cooked rice or with naan bread provides complex carbohydrates and fiber, helping to regulate blood sugar levels and provide sustained energy. Overall, this recipe is a delicious and satisfying option for a balanced meal.

Beef and Broccoli Stir-Fry

Recipe:

Prep Time: 15 minutes
Cook Time: 15 minutes
Number of Servings: 4

Ingredients:

- 1 pound flank steak, thinly sliced against the grain
- ¼ cup low-sodium soy sauce (or tamari for gluten-free option)
- 2 tablespoons hoisin sauce
- 2 tablespoons oyster sauce
- 1 tablespoon rice vinegar
- 1 tablespoon cornstarch
- 1 tablespoon olive oil
- 2 cloves garlic, minced
- 1 tablespoon grated ginger
- 2 cups broccoli florets
- 1 red bell pepper, sliced
- ½ cup sliced carrots
- Cooked rice or noodles, for serving

Instructions:

1. In a small bowl, whisk together the low-sodium soy sauce, hoisin sauce, oyster sauce, rice vinegar, and cornstarch. Set aside.
2. Heat olive oil in a large skillet or wok over medium-high heat.
3. Add minced garlic and grated ginger to the skillet and cook for 1 minute, until fragrant.
4. Add thinly sliced flank steak to the skillet and cook until browned on all sides, about 2-3 minutes. Remove the steak from the skillet and set aside.
5. In the same skillet, add broccoli florets, sliced red bell pepper, and sliced carrots. Stir-fry for 3-4 minutes, until the vegetables are crisp-tender.
6. Return the cooked steak to the skillet.
7. Pour the sauce mixture over the steak and vegetables in the skillet. Stir well to coat everything evenly.
8. Cook for an additional 2-3 minutes, until the sauce has thickened and the steak is heated through.
9. Serve the beef and broccoli stir-fry hot over cooked rice or noodles.

Health Benefits:-

This Beef and Broccoli Stir-Fry is a nutritious and flavorful option for individuals with diabetes. Flank steak is a lean protein source that helps regulate blood sugar levels and promotes satiety. Broccoli, red bell pepper, and carrots provide vitamins, minerals, and antioxidants, supporting overall health and blood sugar control. Low-sodium soy sauce, hoisin sauce, and oyster sauce add flavor to the dish without adding extra sodium or sugar. Serving the stir-fry over cooked rice or noodles provides complex carbohydrates and fiber, helping to regulate blood sugar levels and provide sustained energy. Overall, this recipe is a delicious and satisfying option for a balanced meal.

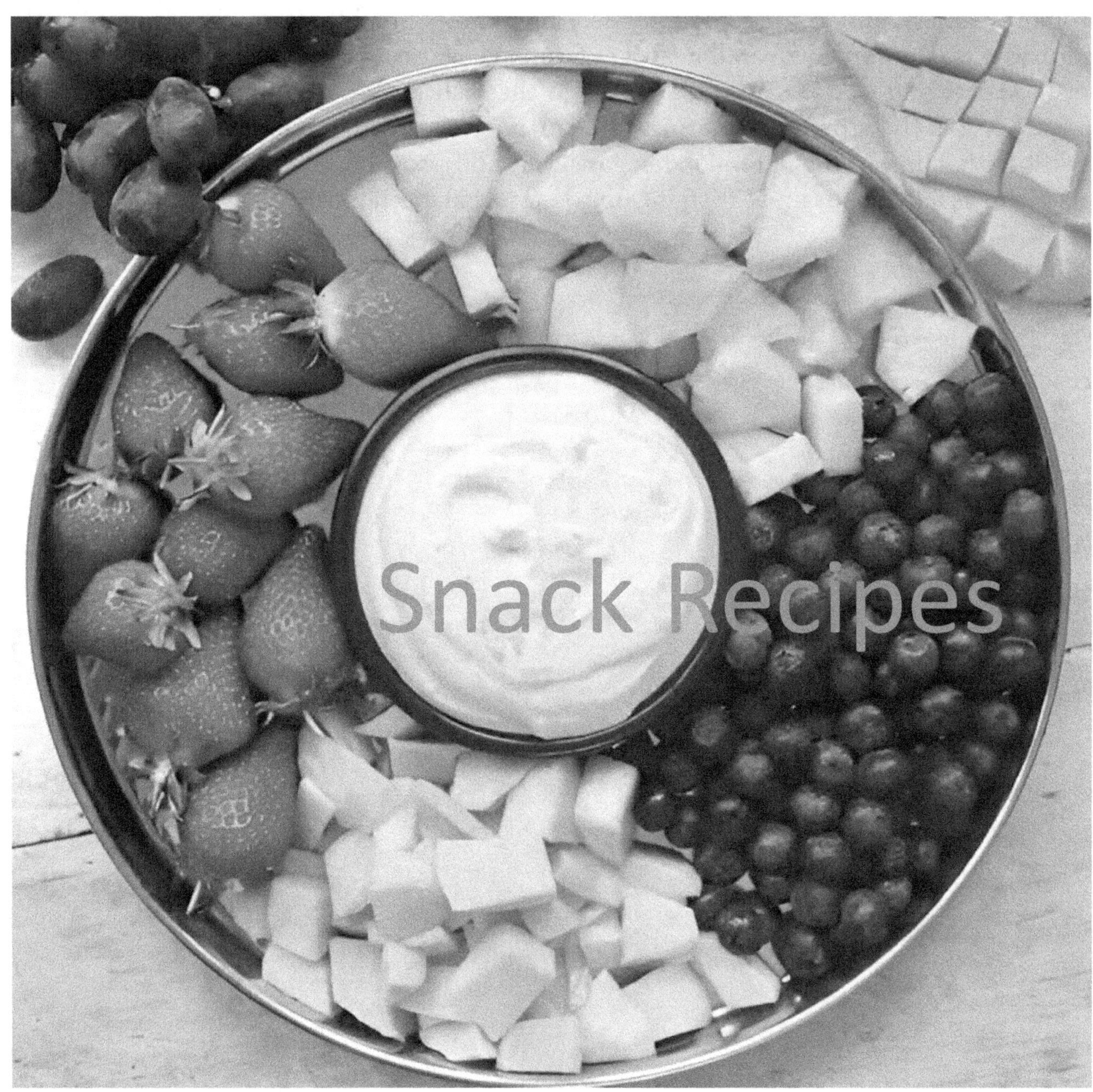
Snack Recipes

Veggie Sticks with Hummus

Recipe :

Prep Time: 10 minutes
Cook Time: 0 minutes
Number of Servings: 4

Ingredients:

- 2 large carrots, peeled and cut into sticks
- 2 celery stalks, cut into sticks
- 1 red bell pepper, cut into strips
- 1 yellow bell pepper, cut into strips
- 1 cucumber, cut into sticks
- 1 cup cherry tomatoes
- 1 cup hummus

Instructions:

1. Wash and prepare all the vegetables as described.
2. Arrange the carrot sticks, celery sticks, red bell pepper strips, yellow bell pepper strips, cucumber sticks, and cherry tomatoes on a serving platter or individual plates.
3. Place the hummus in a serving bowl and place it alongside the vegetable sticks.
4. Serve the veggie sticks with hummus immediately as a nutritious and delicious snack or appetizer.

Health Benefits:-

This Veggie Sticks with Hummus recipe is a healthy and satisfying option for individuals with diabetes. The variety of colorful vegetables provides essential vitamins, minerals, and antioxidants, supporting overall health and blood sugar control. Carrots are rich in beta-carotene, celery is low in calories and high in fiber, bell peppers are high in vitamin C, cucumber is hydrating and low in calories, and cherry tomatoes are rich in vitamins and antioxidants. Hummus is made from chickpeas, which are a good source of protein and fiber, helping to regulate blood sugar levels and promote satiety. Overall, this snack is a nutritious and convenient option for individuals with diabetes.

Greek Yogurt Dip with Fresh Fruit

Recipe :

Prep Time: 10 minutes
Cook Time: 0 minutes
Number of Servings: 4

Ingredients:

- 1 cup plain Greek yogurt
- 1 tablespoon honey (optional, adjust to taste)
- ½ teaspoon vanilla extract
- Assorted fresh fruits (such as strawberries, blueberries, grapes, apple slices, and banana slices) for dipping

Instructions:

1. In a small mixing bowl, combine the plain Greek yogurt, honey (if using), and vanilla extract. Stir until well combined.
2. Wash and prepare the assorted fresh fruits as desired.
3. Arrange the fresh fruit on a serving platter or individual plates.
4. Serve the Greek yogurt dip alongside the fresh fruit for dipping.

Health Benefits:-

This Greek Yogurt Dip with Fresh Fruit is a healthy and refreshing option for individuals with diabetes. Greek yogurt is high in protein and low in carbohydrates, which helps regulate blood sugar levels and promotes satiety. It also provides probiotics, which support gut health. Honey (if using) adds sweetness to the dip without adding extra sugar, and vanilla extract adds flavor. Assorted fresh fruits provide essential vitamins, minerals, and antioxidants, supporting overall health and blood sugar control. Strawberries are high in vitamin C and fiber, blueberries are rich in antioxidants, grapes provide natural sweetness, apple slices are high in fiber, and banana slices are rich in potassium. Overall, this snack is a nutritious and satisfying option for individuals with diabetes.

Trail Mix with Nuts and Seeds

Recipe:

Prep Time: 5 minutes
Cook Time: 0 minutes
Number of Servings: 8

Ingredients:

- 1 cup almonds
- 1 cup walnuts
- 1 cup cashews
- 1 cup pumpkin seeds
- 1 cup sunflower seeds
- ½ cup dried cranberries
- ½ cup dark chocolate chips (optional)

Instructions:

1. In a large mixing bowl, combine the almonds, walnuts, cashews, pumpkin seeds, sunflower seeds, dried cranberries, and dark chocolate chips (if using).
2. Mix well to combine.
3. Store the trail mix in an airtight container or individual portion-sized bags for convenient snacking.

Health Benefits:-

This Trail Mix with Nuts and Seeds is a nutritious and convenient snack option for individuals with diabetes. Almonds, walnuts, cashews, pumpkin seeds, and sunflower seeds are all rich in healthy fats, protein, and fiber, which help regulate blood sugar levels and promote satiety. Dried cranberries add natural sweetness and provide vitamins, minerals, and antioxidants. Dark chocolate chips (if using) add a touch of sweetness and provide additional antioxidants. This trail mix is a balanced and satisfying snack that provides essential nutrients and energy for individuals with diabetes.

Cottage Cheese with Pineapple

Recipe :

Prep Time: 5 minutes
Cook Time: 0 minutes
Number of Servings: 2

Ingredients:

- 1 cup cottage cheese
- 1 cup fresh pineapple chunks

Instructions:

1. In a serving bowl, place the cottage cheese.
2. Top the cottage cheese with fresh pineapple chunks.
3. Serve immediately as a refreshing and nutritious snack or breakfast option.

Health Benefits:-

This Cottage Cheese with Pineapple is a simple and nutritious snack or breakfast option for individuals with diabetes. Cottage cheese is low in carbohydrates and high in protein, which helps regulate blood sugar levels and promotes satiety. It also provides calcium and other essential nutrients. Fresh pineapple chunks add natural sweetness and provide vitamins, minerals, and antioxidants, including vitamin C and bromelain, which have anti-inflammatory properties. This snack is a delicious and satisfying option for individuals with diabetes.

Apple Slices with Almond Butter

Recipe :

Prep Time: 5 minutes
Cook Time: 0 minutes
Number of Servings: 2

Ingredients:

- 1 large apple, cored and sliced
- 2 tablespoons almond butter

Instructions:

1. Slice the apple into thin slices and remove the core.
2. Spread almond butter on each apple slice.
3. Arrange the apple slices on a serving plate.
4. Serve immediately as a delicious and nutritious snack or breakfast option.

Health Benefits:-

This Apple Slices with Almond Butter recipe is a nutritious and satisfying snack or breakfast option for individuals with diabetes. Apples are low in calories and high in fiber, which helps regulate blood sugar levels and promotes satiety. They also provide vitamins, minerals, and antioxidants, including vitamin C and polyphenols. Almond butter is rich in healthy fats, protein, and fiber, which help regulate blood sugar levels and promote satiety. It also provides essential nutrients, including vitamin E and magnesium. This snack is a delicious and wholesome option for individuals with diabetes.

Popcorn with Herbs and Parmesan

Recipe:

Prep Time: 5 minutes
Cook Time: 5 minutes
Number of Servings: 4

Ingredients:

- ½ cup popcorn kernels
- 2 tablespoons olive oil
- 2 tablespoons grated Parmesan cheese
- 1 teaspoon dried Italian herbs (such as oregano, basil, and thyme)
- Salt, to taste

Instructions:

1. Heat olive oil in a large pot over medium heat.
2. Add popcorn kernels to the pot and cover with a lid.
3. Cook, shaking the pot occasionally, until the popping slows down, about 3-5 minutes.
4. Remove the pot from heat and let it sit for a minute to allow any remaining kernels to pop.
5. Transfer the popped popcorn to a large mixing bowl.
6. Sprinkle grated Parmesan cheese, dried Italian herbs, and salt over the popcorn.
7. Toss the popcorn gently to coat evenly with the seasonings.
8. Serve immediately as a flavorful and satisfying snack.

Health Benefits:-

This Popcorn with Herbs and Parmesan recipe is a tasty and satisfying snack option for individuals with diabetes. Popcorn is a whole grain that is low in calories and high in fiber, which helps regulate blood sugar levels and promotes satiety. Olive oil adds heart-healthy monounsaturated fats, while Parmesan cheese provides flavor and a source of calcium. Dried Italian herbs add flavor without adding extra calories or carbohydrates. This snack is a delicious and wholesome option for individuals with diabetes.

Mini Cheese and Veggie Kabobs

Recipe:

Prep Time: 15 minutes
Cook Time: 0 minutes
Number of Servings: 4

Ingredients:

- 16 cherry tomatoes
- 16 mini fresh mozzarella balls (bocconcini)
- 16 small basil leaves
- 16 black olives
- 16 small cucumber chunks
- 16 toothpicks or mini skewers

Instructions:

1. Assemble the kabobs by threading one cherry tomato, one mini mozzarella ball, one basil leaf, one black olive, and one cucumber chunk onto each toothpick or mini skewer, in that order.
2. Repeat the process until all ingredients are used and you have 16 mini cheese and veggie kabobs.
3. Arrange the kabobs on a serving platter and serve immediately as a tasty and colorful appetizer or snack.

Health Benefits:-

These Mini Cheese and Veggie Kabobs are a nutritious and flavorful snack or appetizer option for individuals with diabetes. Cherry tomatoes are low in calories and high in vitamin C and antioxidants, while mini fresh mozzarella balls provide calcium and protein. Basil leaves add flavor and essential nutrients, while black olives provide healthy fats. Cucumber chunks are hydrating and low in calories, adding crunch to the kabobs. This snack is a delicious and wholesome option for individuals with diabetes.

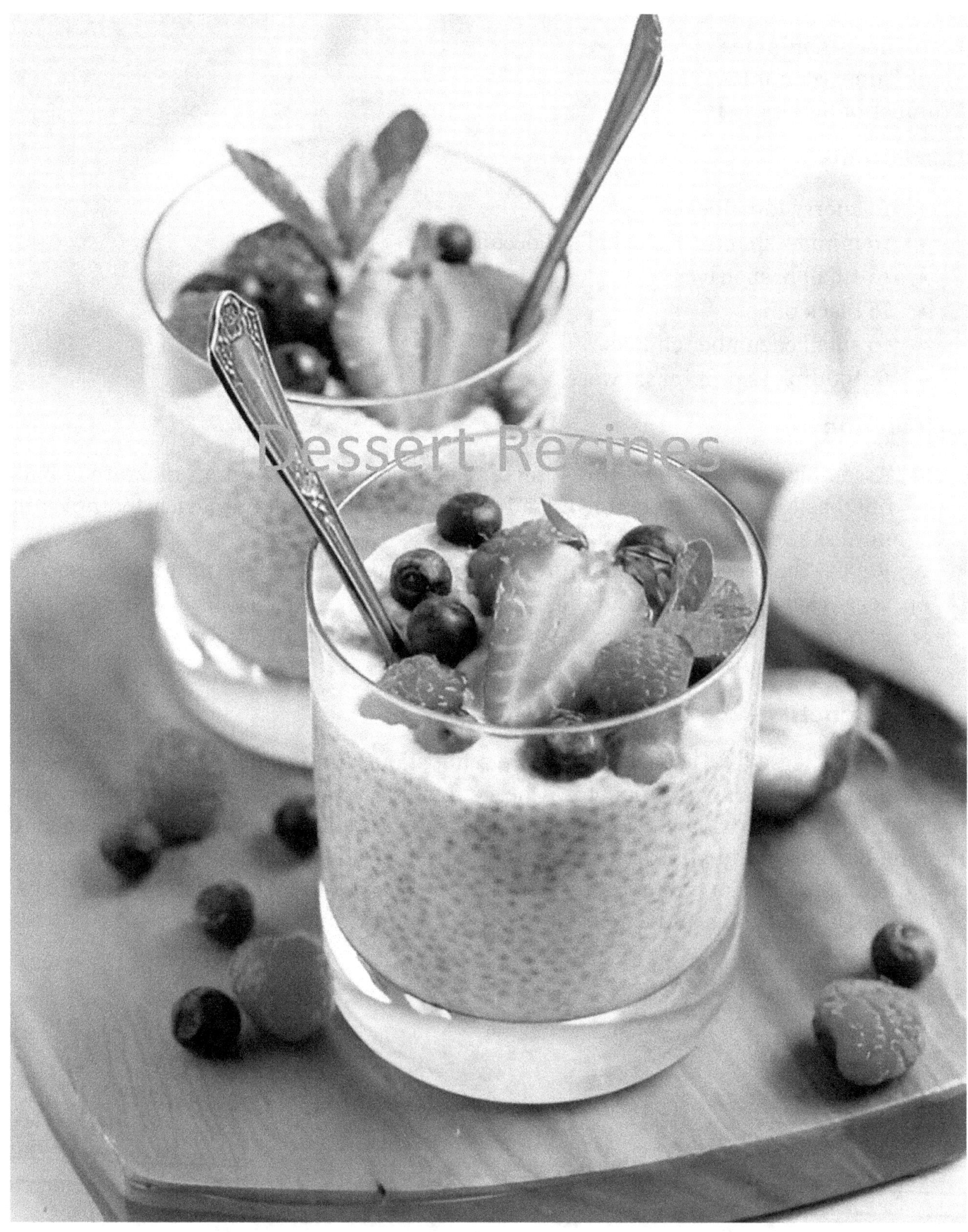
Dessert Recipes

Baked Apples with Cinnamon and Walnuts

Recipe:

Prep Time: 10 minutes
Cook Time: 30 minutes
Number of Servings: 4

Ingredients:

- 4 apples (such as Honeycrisp or Granny Smith)
- 2 tablespoons unsalted butter, melted
- 2 tablespoons brown sugar or sweetener of choice
- 1 teaspoon ground cinnamon
- ¼ cup chopped walnuts
- Vanilla Greek yogurt or whipped cream, for serving (optional)

Instructions:

1. Preheat the oven to 375°F (190°C). Grease a baking dish large enough to hold the apples.
2. Wash and core the apples, leaving the bottoms intact. Place the apples in the prepared baking dish.
3. In a small bowl, mix together the melted butter, brown sugar, ground cinnamon, and chopped walnuts.
4. Stuff each cored apple with the buttery cinnamon walnut mixture, dividing it evenly among the apples.
5. Cover the baking dish with aluminum foil and bake in the preheated oven for 20 minutes.
6. Remove the foil and bake for an additional 10 minutes, or until the apples are tender and the filling is bubbly.
7. Remove from the oven and let the baked apples cool slightly before serving.
8. Serve the baked apples warm, topped with a dollop of vanilla Greek yogurt or whipped cream if desired.

Health Benefits:-

These Baked Apples with Cinnamon and Walnuts are a delicious and comforting dessert option for individuals with diabetes. Apples are rich in fiber and antioxidants, which help regulate blood sugar levels and support overall health. Walnuts provide heart-healthy omega-3 fatty acids and protein, while cinnamon adds flavor and may help improve insulin sensitivity. This recipe is a healthier alternative to traditional baked desserts, as it contains no refined sugars and is naturally sweetened with brown sugar and apples. Serve these baked apples warm with a dollop of vanilla Greek yogurt or whipped cream for a satisfying and guilt-free treat.

Dark Chocolate Avocado Mousse

Recipe:

Prep Time: 10 minutes
Cook Time: 0 minutes
Chill Time: 2 hours
Number of Servings: 4

Ingredients:

- 2 ripe avocados, peeled and pitted
- ¼ cup unsweetened cocoa powder
- ¼ cup maple syrup or sweetener of choice
- 1 teaspoon vanilla extract
- ¼ cup almond milk or milk of choice
- 3 ounces dark chocolate (at least 70% cocoa), melted
- Optional toppings: whipped cream, berries, shaved chocolate

Instructions:

1. In a food processor or blender, combine the ripe avocados, unsweetened cocoa powder, maple syrup, vanilla extract, and almond milk.
2. Blend until smooth and creamy, scraping down the sides of the bowl as needed.
3. Add the melted dark chocolate to the avocado mixture and blend again until well combined.
4. Taste the mousse and adjust sweetness if needed by adding more maple syrup.
5. Transfer the mousse to serving dishes or ramekins.
6. Cover and refrigerate for at least 2 hours, or until the mousse is chilled and set.
7. Before serving, garnish with whipped cream, berries, or shaved chocolate if desired.

Health Benefits:-

This Dark Chocolate Avocado Mousse is a decadent and creamy dessert option for individuals with diabetes. Avocados are rich in heart-healthy monounsaturated fats, fiber, and antioxidants, which help regulate blood sugar levels and support overall health. Unsweetened cocoa powder and dark chocolate are low in sugar and high in antioxidants, providing a rich chocolate flavor without adding extra sugars. Maple syrup adds sweetness without causing rapid spikes in blood sugar levels. This mousse is a healthier alternative to traditional chocolate desserts and is perfect for satisfying sweet cravings in a balanced way.

Banana Oatmeal Cookies

Recipe :

Prep Time: 10 minutes
Cook Time: 15 minutes
Number of Servings: 12 cookies

Ingredients:

- 2 ripe bananas, mashed
- 1 cup rolled oats
- ¼ cup unsweetened applesauce
- ¼ cup almond butter or peanut butter
- ¼ cup chopped nuts (such as walnuts or almonds)
- ¼ cup dried cranberries or raisins (optional)
- 1 teaspoon vanilla extract
- 1 teaspoon ground cinnamon
- Pinch of salt

Instructions:

1. Preheat the oven to 350°F (175°C). Line a baking sheet with parchment paper.
2. In a large mixing bowl, combine the mashed bananas, rolled oats, unsweetened applesauce, almond butter or peanut butter, chopped nuts, dried cranberries or raisins (if using), vanilla extract, ground cinnamon, and a pinch of salt.
3. Mix well until all ingredients are thoroughly combined.
4. Drop spoonfuls of the cookie dough onto the prepared baking sheet, spacing them apart.
5. Flatten each cookie slightly with the back of a spoon or fork.
6. Bake in the preheated oven for 12-15 minutes, or until the cookies are golden brown and firm to the touch.
7. Remove from the oven and let the cookies cool on the baking sheet for a few minutes before transferring them to a wire rack to cool completely.
8. Once cooled, store the banana oatmeal cookies in an airtight container at room temperature for up to 3 days.

Health Benefits:-

These Banana Oatmeal Cookies are a delicious and nutritious treat for individuals with diabetes. Bananas are a good source of fiber, potassium, and vitamins, while rolled oats provide complex carbohydrates and fiber, helping to regulate blood sugar levels and promote satiety. Unsweetened applesauce adds moisture and natural sweetness to the cookies without adding extra sugars. Almond butter or peanut butter provides healthy fats and protein, which help stabilize blood sugar levels and keep you feeling full. Chopped nuts and dried cranberries or raisins (if using) add texture, flavor, and additional nutrients. Overall, these cookies are a satisfying and guilt-free snack option for individuals with diabetes.

Coconut Chia Seed Pudding with Berries

Recipe:

Prep Time: 5 minutes
Chill Time: 4 hours or overnight
Number of Servings: 4

Ingredients:

- 1 can (13.5 ounces) coconut milk (full-fat)
- ¼ cup chia seeds
- 2 tablespoons maple syrup or sweetener of choice
- 1 teaspoon vanilla extract
- 1 cup mixed berries (such as strawberries, blueberries, raspberries)

Instructions:-

1. In a mixing bowl, whisk together the coconut milk, chia seeds, maple syrup, and vanilla extract until well combined.
2. Cover the bowl and refrigerate for at least 4 hours or overnight, allowing the chia seeds to absorb the liquid and thicken the pudding.
3. Stir the pudding mixture well before serving to evenly distribute the chia seeds.
4. Divide the coconut chia seed pudding into serving bowls or glasses.
5. Top each serving with a handful of mixed berries.
6. Serve the coconut chia seed pudding with berries chilled as a delicious and nutritious dessert or breakfast option.

Health Benefits:-

This Coconut Chia Seed Pudding with Berries is a creamy and satisfying dessert or breakfast option for individuals with diabetes. Coconut milk is rich in healthy fats and medium-chain triglycerides (MCTs), which provide sustained energy and support blood sugar control. Chia seeds are packed with fiber, omega-3 fatty acids, and antioxidants, helping to regulate blood sugar levels and promote satiety. Maple syrup adds natural sweetness without causing rapid spikes in blood sugar levels. Mixed berries are low in calories and high in fiber, vitamins, minerals, and antioxidants, supporting overall health and blood sugar control. This pudding is a delicious and wholesome option for individuals with diabetes.

Greek Yogurt Bark with Berries and Almonds

Recipe:

Prep Time: 10 minutes
Freeze Time: 2 hours
Number of Servings: 6

Ingredients:

- 2 cups plain Greek yogurt
- 2 tablespoons honey or maple syrup
- 1 teaspoon vanilla extract
- ¼ cup sliced almonds
- ¼ cup mixed berries (such as strawberries, blueberries, raspberries)

Instructions:

1. In a mixing bowl, combine the plain Greek yogurt, honey or maple syrup, and vanilla extract. Mix until well combined.
2. Line a baking sheet with parchment paper.
3. Pour the Greek yogurt mixture onto the prepared baking sheet, spreading it out evenly with a spatula to create a thin layer.
4. Sprinkle sliced almonds and mixed berries over the Greek yogurt mixture, pressing them down lightly to adhere.
5. Place the baking sheet in the freezer and freeze for at least 2 hours, or until the yogurt bark is firm.
6. Once frozen, remove the baking sheet from the freezer and break the yogurt bark into pieces using your hands or a knife.
7. Serve the Greek yogurt bark with berries and almonds immediately as a refreshing and nutritious snack or dessert.

Health Benefits:-

This Greek Yogurt Bark with Berries and Almonds is a delicious and nutritious snack or dessert option for individuals with diabetes. Greek yogurt is high in protein and low in carbohydrates, which helps regulate blood sugar levels and promotes satiety. It also provides probiotics, which support gut health. Honey or maple syrup adds sweetness without causing rapid spikes in blood sugar levels. Sliced almonds are rich in healthy fats, protein, and fiber, while mixed berries provide vitamins, minerals, and antioxidants. This yogurt bark is a satisfying and guilt-free treat for individuals with diabetes.

Pumpkin Spice Energy Bites

Recipe:

Prep Time: 10 minutes
Chill Time: 30 minutes
Number of Servings: 12-15 bites

Ingredients:

- 1 cup rolled oats
- ½ cup pumpkin puree
- ¼ cup almond butter or peanut butter
- ¼ cup honey or maple syrup
- 1 teaspoon pumpkin pie spice
- ½ teaspoon vanilla extract
- ¼ cup chopped nuts (such as pecans or walnuts)
- ¼ cup mini chocolate chips (optional)
- Additional rolled oats for rolling (optional)

Instructions:

1. In a mixing bowl, combine the rolled oats, pumpkin puree, almond butter or peanut butter, honey or maple syrup, pumpkin pie spice, and vanilla extract. Mix until well combined.
2. Stir in the chopped nuts and mini chocolate chips (if using) until evenly distributed throughout the mixture.
3. Cover the bowl and refrigerate the mixture for at least 30 minutes to allow it to firm up.
4. Once chilled, use a tablespoon or cookie scoop to portion out the mixture and roll it into bite-sized balls.
5. If desired, roll the energy bites in additional rolled oats for added texture.
6. Place the energy bites on a parchment-lined baking sheet and refrigerate for an additional 30 minutes to set.
7. Once set, transfer the pumpkin spice energy bites to an airtight container and store them in the refrigerator for up to one week.

Health Benefits:-

These Pumpkin Spice Energy Bites are a nutritious and delicious snack option for individuals with diabetes. Rolled oats provide complex carbohydrates and fiber, helping to regulate blood sugar levels and promote satiety. Pumpkin puree is rich in fiber, vitamins, and minerals, including vitamin A and potassium. Almond butter or peanut butter provides healthy fats and protein, which help stabilize blood sugar levels and keep you feeling full. Honey or maple syrup adds natural sweetness without causing rapid spikes in blood sugar levels. Chopped nuts and mini chocolate chips (if using) add texture and flavor, while also providing additional nutrients. These energy bites are a convenient and satisfying snack for individuals with diabetes.

Berry Crumble Parfait

Recipe :

Prep Time: 15 minutes
Cook Time: 30 minutes
Chill Time: 1 hour (optional)
Number of Servings: 4

Ingredients :

- o 2 cups mixed berries (such as strawberries, blueberries, raspberries)
  - o 2 tablespoons maple syrup or sweetener of choice
  - o 1 tablespoon lemon juice
  - o 1 tablespoon cornstarch
- Ingredients for Crumble Topping:
  - o ½ cup rolled oats
  - o ¼ cup almond flour or whole wheat flour
  - o ¼ cup chopped nuts (such as almonds or walnuts)
  - o 2 tablespoons coconut oil or unsalted butter, melted
  - o 2 tablespoons maple syrup or sweetener of choice
  - o ½ teaspoon ground cinnamon
- Ingredients for Parfait Assembly:
  - o 2 cups Greek yogurt
  - o Honey or maple syrup, to taste (optional)
  - o Fresh berries for garnish (optional)

Instructions:

1. Berry Filling:
1. Preheat the oven to 350°F (175°C). Grease a baking dish.
2. In a mixing bowl, combine the mixed berries, maple syrup, lemon juice, and cornstarch. Mix until the berries are evenly coated.
3. Transfer the berry mixture to the prepared baking dish and spread it out evenly.
2. Crumble Topping:-
1. In a separate mixing bowl, combine the rolled oats, almond flour or whole wheat flour, chopped nuts, melted coconut oil or unsalted butter, maple syrup, and ground cinnamon. Mix until the ingredients are well combined and crumbly.
2. Sprinkle the crumble topping evenly over the berry mixture in the baking dish.
3. Bake:-
1. Bake in the preheated oven for 25-30 minutes, or until the berry filling is bubbling and the crumble topping is golden brown.
2. Remove from the oven and let the berry crumble cool slightly.

3. Parfait Assembly:-
1. In serving glasses or bowls, layer Greek yogurt, a spoonful of the warm berry crumble, and another layer of Greek yogurt.
2. Drizzle honey or maple syrup over the yogurt layers if desired.
3. Repeat the layers until the glasses or bowls are filled.
4. Garnish with fresh berries if desired.
5. Serve the berry crumble parfait immediately, or chill in the refrigerator for 1 hour before serving for a refreshing treat.

Health Benefits:-

This Berry Crumble Parfait is a delightful and nutritious dessert option for individuals with diabetes. Mixed berries are low in calories and high in fiber, vitamins, and antioxidants, helping to regulate blood sugar levels and support overall health. Rolled oats provide complex carbohydrates and fiber, which promote satiety and help stabilize blood sugar levels. Almond flour or whole wheat flour adds texture and nutrients, while chopped nuts provide healthy fats and protein. Greek yogurt is rich in protein and probiotics, which support gut health and help regulate blood sugar levels. Honey or maple syrup adds natural sweetness without causing rapid spikes in blood sugar levels. This berry crumble parfait is a delicious and satisfying treat for individuals with diabetes.

Chocolate Protein Smoothie

Recipe:

Prep Time: 5 minutes
Number of Servings: 1

Ingredients:

- 1 cup unsweetened almond milk or milk of choice
- 1 scoop chocolate protein powder
- 1 tablespoon unsweetened cocoa powder
- ½ frozen banana
- 1 tablespoon almond butter or peanut butter
- ½ teaspoon vanilla extract
- ½ cup ice cubes
- Optional: 1 tablespoon chia seeds or flaxseeds for added fiber and omega-3 fatty acids

Instructions:

1. In a blender, combine the unsweetened almond milk, chocolate protein powder, unsweetened cocoa powder, frozen banana, almond butter or peanut butter, vanilla extract, and ice cubes.
2. If using, add chia seeds or flaxseeds for added fiber and omega-3 fatty acids.
3. Blend on high speed until smooth and creamy, scraping down the sides of the blender as needed.
4. Taste the smoothie and adjust sweetness or thickness by adding more protein powder, cocoa powder, or almond milk if desired.
5. Pour the chocolate protein smoothie into a glass and serve immediately.

Health Benefits:-

This Chocolate Protein Smoothie is a delicious and nutritious breakfast or post-workout option for individuals with diabetes. Unsweetened almond milk is low in calories and carbohydrates, making it a suitable base for individuals monitoring their blood sugar levels. Chocolate protein powder provides protein to help stabilize blood sugar levels and promote muscle recovery. Unsweetened cocoa powder adds rich chocolate flavor without adding extra sugars. Frozen banana adds natural sweetness and creamy texture, while almond butter or peanut butter adds healthy fats and protein. Chia seeds or flaxseeds (optional) provide fiber and omega-3 fatty acids, which support gut health and cardiovascular health. This chocolate protein smoothie is a satisfying and energizing option for individuals with diabetes.

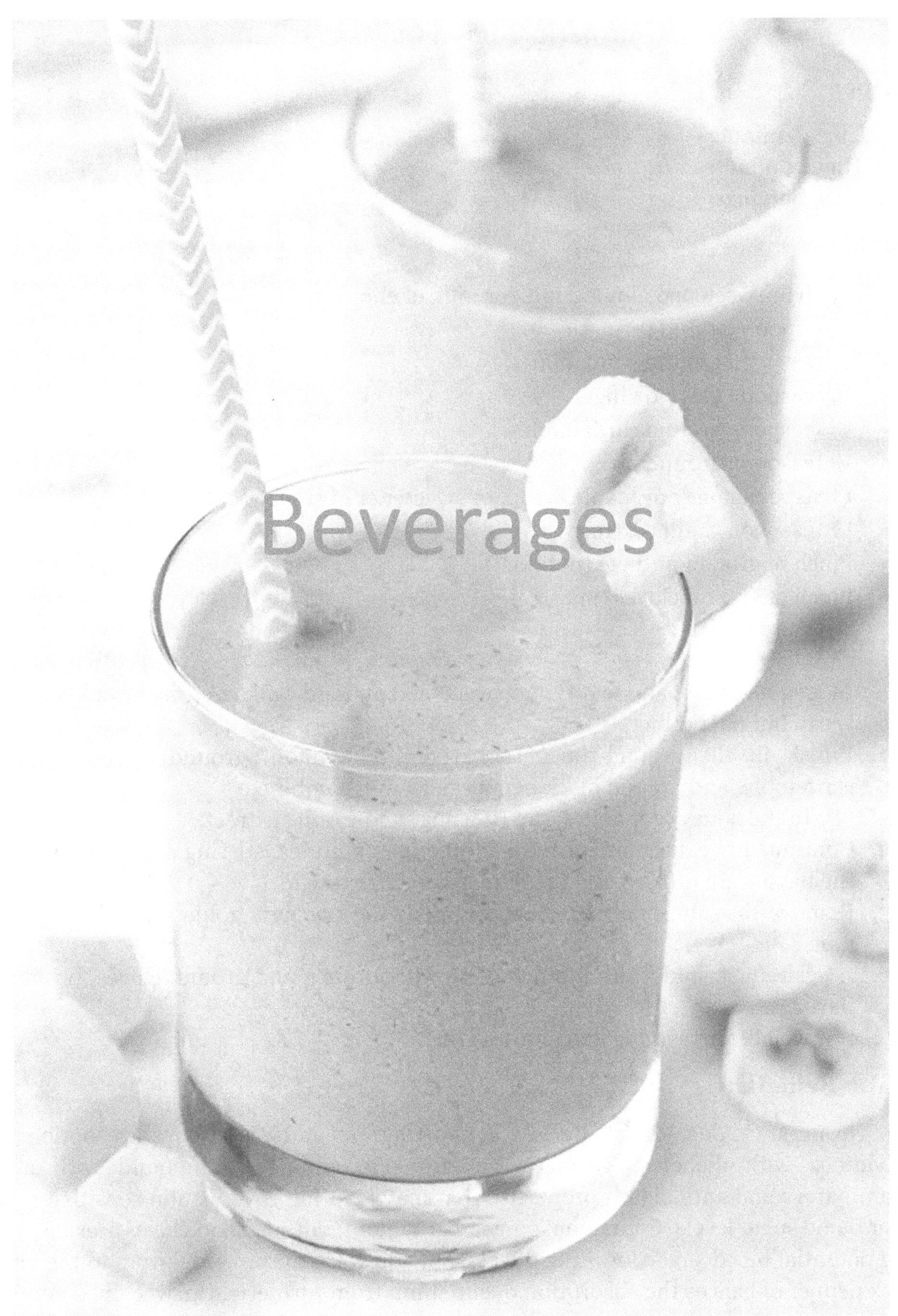
Beverages

Turmeric Golden Milk Latte

Recipe:

Prep Time: 5 minutes
Cook Time: 5 minutes
Number of Servings: 1

Ingredients:

- 1 cup unsweetened almond milk or milk of choice
- 1 teaspoon ground turmeric
- ½ teaspoon ground cinnamon
- ¼ teaspoon ground ginger
- ¼ teaspoon ground cardamom
- ¼ teaspoon ground black pepper
- 1 teaspoon honey or maple syrup, or sweetener of choice (optional)
- ½ teaspoon vanilla extract
- Pinch of ground nutmeg (optional)
- Pinch of ground cloves (optional)

Instructions:

1. In a small saucepan, heat the unsweetened almond milk over medium heat until warm but not boiling.
2. Whisk in the ground turmeric, ground cinnamon, ground ginger, ground cardamom, and ground black pepper until well combined.
3. Stir in the honey or maple syrup (if using) and vanilla extract.
4. Continue to heat the mixture for another 2-3 minutes, stirring occasionally, until the flavors are infused and the latte is heated through.
5. Remove the saucepan from heat and pour the turmeric golden milk latte into a mug.
6. If desired, sprinkle with a pinch of ground nutmeg and ground cloves for added flavor.
7. Stir well before serving and enjoy warm.

Health Benefits:-

This Turmeric Golden Milk Latte is a comforting and nutritious beverage option for individuals with diabetes. Turmeric contains curcumin, a compound with anti-inflammatory and antioxidant properties that may help improve insulin sensitivity and lower blood sugar levels. Cinnamon, ginger, cardamom, nutmeg, and cloves are all spices with potential blood sugar-lowering effects and add warm, aromatic flavors to the latte. Black pepper enhances the absorption of curcumin from turmeric. Unsweetened almond milk is low in calories and carbohydrates, making it a suitable base for individuals monitoring their blood sugar levels. Honey or maple syrup can be added for sweetness, but individuals with diabetes may choose to omit or use a sugar-free sweetener. Overall, this turmeric golden milk latte is a delicious and healthful option for individuals with diabetes.

Berry Blast Protein Shake

Recipe:

Prep Time: 5 minutes
Number of Servings: 1

Ingredients:

- 1 cup unsweetened almond milk or milk of choice
- 1 scoop vanilla or mixed berry-flavored protein powder
- ½ cup mixed berries (such as strawberries, blueberries, raspberries)
- ½ frozen banana
- 1 tablespoon almond butter or peanut butter
- Optional: 1 tablespoon chia seeds or flaxseeds for added fiber and omega-3 fatty acids
- Optional: 1 teaspoon honey or maple syrup, or sweetener of choice (if additional sweetness is desired)

Instructions:

1. In a blender, combine the unsweetened almond milk, vanilla or mixed berry-flavored protein powder, mixed berries, frozen banana, almond butter or peanut butter, and optional chia seeds or flaxseeds.
2. If additional sweetness is desired, add honey or maple syrup or sweetener of choice.
3. Blend on high speed until smooth and creamy, scraping down the sides of the blender as needed.
4. Taste the protein shake and adjust sweetness or thickness by adding more protein powder, berries, or almond milk if desired.
5. Pour the Berry Blast Protein Shake into a glass and serve immediately.

Health Benefits:-

This Berry Blast Protein Shake is a delicious and nutritious breakfast or post-workout option for individuals with diabetes. Unsweetened almond milk is low in calories and carbohydrates, making it a suitable base for individuals monitoring their blood sugar levels. Vanilla or mixed berry-flavored protein powder provides protein to help stabilize blood sugar levels and promote muscle recovery. Mixed berries are low in calories and high in fiber, vitamins, and antioxidants, helping to regulate blood sugar levels and support overall health. Frozen banana adds natural sweetness and creamy texture, while almond butter or peanut butter adds healthy fats and protein. Chia seeds or flaxseeds (optional) provide fiber and omega-3 fatty acids, which support gut health and cardiovascular health. Overall, this Berry Blast Protein Shake is a satisfying and energizing option for individuals with diabetes.

Green Smoothie with Spinach and Mango

Recipe:

Prep Time: 5 minutes
Number of Servings: 1

Ingredients:

- 1 cup unsweetened almond milk or milk of choice
- 1 cup fresh spinach leaves
- ½ cup frozen mango chunks
- ½ frozen banana
- 1 tablespoon almond butter or peanut butter
- 1 tablespoon chia seeds or flaxseeds (optional)
- Optional: 1 teaspoon honey or maple syrup, or sweetener of choice (if additional sweetness is desired)

Instructions:

1. In a blender, combine the unsweetened almond milk, fresh spinach leaves, frozen mango chunks, frozen banana, almond butter or peanut butter, and optional chia seeds or flaxseeds.
2. If additional sweetness is desired, add honey or maple syrup or sweetener of choice.
3. Blend on high speed until smooth and creamy, scraping down the sides of the blender as needed.
4. Taste the smoothie and adjust sweetness or thickness by adding more mango chunks, banana, or almond milk if desired.
5. Pour the Green Smoothie with Spinach and Mango into a glass and serve immediately.

Health Benefits:-

This Green Smoothie with Spinach and Mango is a delicious and nutritious breakfast or snack option for individuals with diabetes. Unsweetened almond milk is low in calories and carbohydrates, making it a suitable base for individuals monitoring their blood sugar levels. Spinach is low in calories and carbohydrates and high in vitamins, minerals, and antioxidants, including vitamin K, vitamin A, and folate. Mango is low in calories and high in fiber, vitamins, and antioxidants, including vitamin C and vitamin A. Frozen banana adds natural sweetness and creamy texture, while almond butter or peanut butter adds healthy fats and protein. Chia seeds or flaxseeds (optional) provide fiber and omega-3 fatty acids, which support gut health and cardiovascular health. Overall, this Green

Smoothie with Spinach and Mango is a refreshing and healthful option for individuals with diabetes.

Iced Herbal Tea with Lemon and Mint

Recipe :

Prep Time: 5 minutes
Chill Time: 2 hours
 Number of Servings: 4

Ingredients:

- 4 cups water
- 4 herbal tea bags (such as chamomile, peppermint, or hibiscus)
- 1 lemon, thinly sliced
- ¼ cup fresh mint leaves
- Optional: honey or sweetener of choice, to taste
- Ice cubes, for serving

Instructions:

1. Bring the water to a boil in a medium saucepan.
2. Remove the saucepan from heat and add the herbal tea bags to the water.
3. Steep the tea bags in the hot water for 5-10 minutes, depending on desired strength.
4. Remove the tea bags from the water and discard.
5. Allow the tea to cool to room temperature, then transfer it to a pitcher or large glass jar.
6. Add the thinly sliced lemon and fresh mint leaves to the pitcher or jar.
7. If desired, sweeten the tea with honey or sweetener of choice, stirring until dissolved.
8. Cover the pitcher or jar and refrigerate the tea for at least 2 hours, or until well chilled.
9. When ready to serve, fill glasses with ice cubes and pour the chilled herbal tea over the ice.
10. Garnish each glass with a sprig of fresh mint and a slice of lemon, if desired.
11. Stir the iced herbal tea with lemon and mint before serving.

Health Benefits:-

This Iced Herbal Tea with Lemon and Mint is a refreshing and hydrating beverage option for individuals with diabetes. Herbal teas like chamomile, peppermint, and hibiscus are naturally caffeine-free and can have various health benefits, including promoting relaxation, digestion, and hydration. Lemon adds a bright and citrusy flavor to the tea, while also providing vitamin C and antioxidants. Fresh mint leaves add a refreshing and cooling element to the tea, while also aiding in digestion. This iced herbal tea is a flavorful and healthful option for staying hydrated and enjoying a refreshing beverage on a hot day.

Cucumber Mint Infused Water

Recipe:

Prep Time: 5 minutes
Chill Time: 1 hour
Number of Servings: 4

Ingredients:

- 4 cups water
- 1 cucumber, thinly sliced
- ¼ cup fresh mint leaves
- Optional: 1 lemon, thinly sliced

Instructions:

1. In a pitcher or large glass jar, combine the water, thinly sliced cucumber, and fresh mint leaves.
2. If using, add the thinly sliced lemon to the pitcher or jar.
3. Stir the ingredients to mix well.
4. Cover the pitcher or jar and refrigerate the cucumber mint infused water for at least 1 hour to allow the flavors to meld.
5. When ready to serve, fill glasses with ice cubes.
6. Pour the chilled cucumber mint infused water into the glasses, making sure to include some cucumber slices and mint leaves in each glass.
7. Stir the infused water before serving to distribute the flavors evenly.
8. Garnish each glass with a sprig of fresh mint, if desired.
9. Serve the cucumber mint infused water chilled and enjoy!

Health Benefits:-

This Cucumber Mint Infused Water is a refreshing and hydrating beverage option for individuals with diabetes. Cucumber is low in calories and carbohydrates and high in water content, making it a hydrating and refreshing addition to water. It also provides vitamins and minerals, including vitamin K and potassium. Fresh mint leaves add a cooling and refreshing flavor to the infused water, while also aiding in digestion. Lemon adds a bright and citrusy flavor to the infused water, as well as providing vitamin C and antioxidants. This cucumber mint infused water is a delicious and healthful way to stay hydrated and enjoy a refreshing beverage throughout the day.

Coconut Water with Lime

Recipe :

Prep Time: 5 minutes
Number of Servings: 1

Ingredients:

- 1 cup coconut water
- ½ lime, juiced
- Ice cubes, for serving (optional)
- Lime slices, for garnish (optional)
- Mint leaves, for garnish (optional)

Instructions:

1. In a glass, combine the coconut water and freshly squeezed lime juice.
2. Stir well to mix the ingredients.
3. If desired, add ice cubes to the glass for a chilled beverage.
4. Garnish the coconut water with lime with lime slices and mint leaves for a refreshing touch.
5. Serve immediately and enjoy!

Health Benefits:-

This Coconut Water with Lime is a refreshing and hydrating beverage option for individuals with diabetes. Coconut water is naturally low in calories and carbohydrates and is a good source of hydration. It also provides electrolytes like potassium, sodium, and magnesium, which help maintain proper fluid balance in the body. Lime juice adds a refreshing citrusy flavor to the coconut water and is rich in vitamin C and antioxidants. This simple and delicious drink is a great way to stay hydrated and enjoy a refreshing beverage on a hot day.

Strawberry Basil Lemonade

Recipe:

Prep Time: 10 minutes
Chill Time: 1 hour
Number of Servings: 4

Ingredients:

- 1 cup fresh strawberries, hulled and sliced
- ¼ cup fresh basil leaves
- ½ cup freshly squeezed lemon juice (about 2-3 lemons)
- ¼ cup honey or maple syrup, or sweetener of choice
- 4 cups water
- Ice cubes, for serving
- Lemon slices and basil leaves, for garnish (optional)

Instructions:

1. In a blender, combine the sliced strawberries, fresh basil leaves, freshly squeezed lemon juice, and honey or maple syrup.
2. Blend until smooth and well combined.
3. Strain the strawberry basil mixture through a fine mesh sieve into a pitcher to remove any seeds or pulp.
4. Discard any solids left in the sieve.
5. Add the water to the pitcher and stir well to mix the ingredients.
6. Cover the pitcher and refrigerate the strawberry basil lemonade for at least 1 hour to chill and allow the flavors to meld.
7. When ready to serve, fill glasses with ice cubes.
8. Pour the chilled strawberry basil lemonade into the glasses.
9. Garnish each glass with a slice of lemon and a sprig of fresh basil, if desired.
10. Serve immediately and enjoy!

Health Benefits:-

This Strawberry Basil Lemonade is a refreshing and hydrating beverage option for individuals with diabetes. Strawberries are low in calories and carbohydrates and high in fiber, vitamins, and antioxidants, including vitamin C and manganese. Basil adds a refreshing and aromatic flavor to the lemonade and is rich in vitamins and minerals, including vitamin K and iron. Lemon juice provides a bright and citrusy flavor to the lemonade and is rich in vitamin C and antioxidants. Honey or maple syrup can be added for sweetness, but individuals with diabetes may choose to omit or use a sugar-free sweetener. This flavorful and healthful drink is a delicious way to stay hydrated and enjoy a refreshing beverage on a hot day.

Pineapple Ginger Smoothie

Recipe:

Prep Time: 5 minutes
Number of Servings: 1
Ingredients:

- 1 cup fresh pineapple chunks
- ½ cup coconut water or water
- ½ banana, frozen
- ½ teaspoon freshly grated ginger
- ½ cup Greek yogurt or coconut yogurt
- Optional: honey or sweetener of choice, to taste
- Ice cubes, for serving (optional)

Instructions:

1. In a blender, combine the fresh pineapple chunks, coconut water or water, frozen banana, freshly grated ginger, and Greek yogurt or coconut yogurt.
2. Blend on high speed until smooth and creamy, scraping down the sides of the blender as needed.
3. If additional sweetness is desired, add honey or sweetener of choice and blend again until well combined.
4. If a colder smoothie is preferred, add ice cubes to the blender and blend until smooth.
5. Pour the Pineapple Ginger Smoothie into a glass and serve immediately.

Health Benefits:-

This Pineapple Ginger Smoothie is a refreshing and nutritious beverage option for individuals with diabetes. Pineapple is low in calories and carbohydrates and high in fiber, vitamins, and minerals, including vitamin C and manganese. It also contains bromelain, an enzyme that may aid in digestion and reduce inflammation. Freshly grated ginger adds a spicy and aromatic flavor to the smoothie and is known for its anti-inflammatory and digestive properties. Coconut water or water provides hydration without added sugars or calories. Greek yogurt or coconut yogurt adds creaminess and protein to the smoothie, helping to stabilize blood sugar levels and promote satiety. This flavorful and healthful smoothie is a delicious way to incorporate pineapple and ginger into your diet while staying hydrated and enjoying a refreshing beverage.

4-Weeks Meal Plan

Here's a 4-week meal plan for individuals with diabetes, incorporating recipes with provided ingredients, instructions, and health benefits:

Week 1:

Day 1:

- Breakfast: Greek Yogurt Parfait with Nuts and Berries
- Lunch: Tuna Salad Lettuce Wraps
- Dinner: Grilled Lemon Herb Chicken with Garlic Roasted Broccoli with Lemon
- Snack: Veggie Sticks with Hummus

Day 2:

- Breakfast: Peanut Butter Banana Toast
- Lunch: Lentil Vegetable Soup
- Dinner: Stuffed Bell Peppers with Quinoa and Ground Turkey
- Snack: Greek Yogurt Dip with Fresh Fruit

Day 3:

- Breakfast: Egg and Avocado Breakfast Wrap
- Lunch: Chicken Caesar Salad
- Dinner: Salmon with Dill Sauce served with Quinoa and Black Bean Salad
- Snack: Trail Mix with Nuts and Seeds

Day 4:

- Breakfast: Greek Yogurt Bark with Berries and Almonds
- Lunch: Caprese Salad with Balsamic Glaze
- Dinner: Beef and Broccoli Stir-Fry
- Snack: Cottage Cheese with Pineapple

Day 5:

- Breakfast: Coconut Chia Seed Pudding with Berries
- Lunch: Vegetable and Chickpea Curry
- Dinner: Spaghetti Squash with Turkey Meatballs and Marinara Sauce
- Snack: Apple Slices with Almond Butter

Day 6:

- Breakfast: Dark Chocolate Avocado Mousse
- Lunch: Turkey and Avocado Wrap
- Dinner: Veggie Sticks with Hummus
- Snack: Popcorn with Herbs and Parmesan

Day 7:

- Breakfast: Banana Oatmeal Cookies
- Lunch: Lentil Vegetable Soup
- Dinner: Baked Cod with Tomato and Basil
- Snack: Greek Yogurt Parfait with Nuts and Berries

Week 2:

Day 1:

- Breakfast: Greek Yogurt Parfait with Nuts and Berries
- Lunch: Chicken and Vegetable Stir-Fry
- Dinner: Lentil Vegetable Soup
- Snack: Veggie Sticks with Hummus

Day 2:

- Breakfast: Peanut Butter Banana Toast
- Lunch: Greek Yogurt Dip with Fresh Fruit
- Dinner: Stuffed Bell Peppers with Quinoa and Ground Turkey
- Snack: Trail Mix with Nuts and Seeds

Day 3:

- Breakfast: Egg and Avocado Breakfast Wrap
- Lunch: Caprese Salad with Balsamic Glaze
- Dinner: Beef and Broccoli Stir-Fry
- Snack: Cottage Cheese with Pineapple

Day 4:

- Breakfast: Greek Yogurt Bark with Berries and Almonds
- Lunch: Turkey and Avocado Wrap
- Dinner: Spaghetti Squash with Turkey Meatballs and Marinara Sauce

- Snack: Apple Slices with Almond Butter

Day 5:

- Breakfast: Coconut Chia Seed Pudding with Berries
- Lunch: Vegetable and Chickpea Curry
- Dinner: Baked Cod with Tomato and Basil
- Snack: Popcorn with Herbs and Parmesan

Day 6:

- Breakfast: Dark Chocolate Avocado Mousse
- Lunch: Tuna Salad Lettuce Wraps
- Dinner: Garlic Roasted Broccoli with Lemon served with Grilled Lemon Herb Chicken
- Snack: Greek Yogurt Parfait with Nuts and Berries

Day 7:

- Breakfast: Banana Oatmeal Cookies
- Lunch: Chicken Caesar Salad
- Dinner: Quinoa and Black Bean Salad
- Snack: Greek Yogurt Dip with Fresh Fruit

Week 3:

Day 1:

- Breakfast: Greek Yogurt Parfait with Nuts and Berries
- Lunch: Chicken and Vegetable Stir-Fry
- Dinner: Lentil Vegetable Soup
- Snack: Veggie Sticks with Hummus

Day 2:

- Breakfast: Peanut Butter Banana Toast

- Lunch: Greek Yogurt Dip with Fresh Fruit
- Dinner: Stuffed Bell Peppers with Quinoa and Ground Turkey
- Snack: Trail Mix with Nuts and Seeds

Day 3:

- Breakfast: Egg and Avocado Breakfast Wrap
- Lunch: Caprese Salad with Balsamic Glaze
- Dinner: Beef and Broccoli Stir-Fry
- Snack: Cottage Cheese with Pineapple

Day 4:

- Breakfast: Greek Yogurt Bark with Berries and Almonds
- Lunch: Turkey and Avocado Wrap
- Dinner: Spaghetti Squash with Turkey Meatballs and Marinara Sauce
- Snack: Apple Slices with Almond Butter

Day 5:

- Breakfast: Coconut Chia Seed Pudding with Berries
- Lunch: Vegetable and Chickpea Curry
- Dinner: Baked Cod with Tomato and Basil
- Snack: Popcorn with Herbs and Parmesan

Day 6:

- Breakfast: Dark Chocolate Avocado Mousse
- Lunch: Tuna Salad Lettuce Wraps
- Dinner: Garlic Roasted Broccoli with Lemon served with Grilled Lemon Herb Chicken
- Snack: Greek Yogurt Parfait with Nuts and Berries

Day 7:

- Breakfast: Banana Oatmeal Cookies
- Lunch: Chicken Caesar Salad

- Dinner: Quinoa and Black Bean Salad
- Snack: Greek Yogurt Dip with Fresh Fruit

Week 4:

Day 1:

- Breakfast: Greek Yogurt Parfait with Nuts and Berries
- Lunch: Chicken and Vegetable Stir-Fry
- Dinner: Lentil Vegetable Soup
- Snack: Veggie Sticks with Hummus

Day 2:

- Breakfast: Peanut Butter Banana Toast
- Lunch: Greek Yogurt Dip with Fresh Fruit
- Dinner: Stuffed Bell Peppers with Quinoa and Ground Turkey
- Snack: Trail Mix with Nuts and Seeds

Day 3:

- Breakfast: Egg and Avocado Breakfast Wrap
- Lunch: Caprese Salad with Balsamic Glaze
- Dinner: Beef and Broccoli Stir-Fry
- Snack: Cottage Cheese with Pineapple

Day 4:

- Breakfast: Greek Yogurt Bark with Berries and Almonds
- Lunch: Turkey and Avocado Wrap
- Dinner: Spaghetti Squash with Turkey Meatballs and Marinara Sauce
- Snack: Apple Slices with Almond Butter

Day 5:

- Breakfast: Coconut Chia Seed Pudding with Berries

- Lunch: Vegetable and Chickpea Curry
- Dinner: Baked Cod with Tomato and Basil
- Snack: Popcorn with Herbs and Parmesan

Day 6:

- Breakfast: Dark Chocolate Avocado Mousse
- Lunch: Tuna Salad Lettuce Wraps
- Dinner: Garlic Roasted Broccoli with Lemon served with Grilled Lemon Herb Chicken
- Snack: Greek Yogurt Parfait with Nuts and Berries

Day 7:

- Breakfast: Banana Oatmeal Cookies
- Lunch: Chicken Caesar Salad
- Dinner: Quinoa and Black Bean Salad
- Snack: Greek Yogurt Dip with Fresh Fruit

Feel free to adjust the meal plan based on individual preferences, dietary needs, and portion sizes. Remember to consult with a healthcare provider or registered dietitian for personalized guidance on managing diabetes through nutrition.

Tips for Meal Planning and Healthy Eating

How to Create Balanced Meals

Creating balanced meals is essential for maintaining overall health and well-being, especially for individuals with diabetes. A balanced meal consists of a variety of nutrients, including carbohydrates, protein, healthy fats, fiber, vitamins, and minerals, in appropriate proportions to support blood sugar control, energy levels, and overall health. Here's a detailed discussion on how to create balanced meals:

1. **Understand Macronutrients:-**

Carbohydrates: Carbohydrates are the body's main source of energy and have the most significant impact on blood sugar levels. Choose complex carbohydrates like whole grains, fruits, vegetables, and legumes, which provide fiber and help regulate blood sugar levels.

Protein: Protein is essential for muscle repair and growth, as well as for maintaining satiety. Include lean sources of protein such as poultry, fish, tofu, legumes, and low-fat dairy products in your meals.

Healthy Fats: Healthy fats are important for heart health and provide sustained energy. Incorporate sources of unsaturated fats like avocados, nuts, seeds, olive oil, and fatty fish (such as salmon and mackerel) into your meals.

Fiber: Fiber aids in digestion, promotes satiety, and helps stabilize blood sugar levels. Include fiber-rich foods like whole grains, fruits, vegetables, nuts, seeds, and legumes in your meals.

2. **Portion Control:**

- Pay attention to portion sizes to avoid overeating and manage blood sugar levels. Use measuring cups, spoons, or visual cues to estimate portion sizes.
- Aim to fill half of your plate with non-starchy vegetables, one-quarter with lean protein, and one-quarter with whole grains or starchy vegetables.
- Be mindful of portion sizes for carbohydrate-rich foods, especially if you're counting carbohydrates to manage blood sugar levels.

3. **Include a Variety of Foods:**

- Incorporate a variety of nutrient-dense foods from all food groups to ensure you're getting a wide range of essential nutrients.
- Choose a rainbow of colorful fruits and vegetables to maximize nutrient intake and provide antioxidants that support overall health.

- Include sources of lean protein, such as poultry, fish, tofu, legumes, and low-fat dairy products, to meet your protein needs.
- Incorporate whole grains like brown rice, quinoa, whole wheat bread, and oats for fiber and sustained energy.

4. **Balance Your Plate:**

- Aim to create balanced meals that contain a combination of carbohydrates, protein, and healthy fats to support blood sugar control and provide sustained energy.
- Choose high-fiber carbohydrates that have a lower glycemic index to help prevent rapid spikes in blood sugar levels.
- Include lean sources of protein and healthy fats to promote satiety and stabilize blood sugar levels.
- Incorporate a variety of foods into your meals to ensure you're meeting your nutritional needs and enjoying a diverse diet.

5. **Consider Meal Timing and Frequency:**

- Space out your meals evenly throughout the day to help manage blood sugar levels and prevent spikes and crashes.
- Aim to eat every 3-4 hours to maintain stable energy levels and prevent overeating.
- Consider including snacks between meals if needed to prevent hunger and maintain blood sugar control.

6. **Hydration:**

- Stay hydrated by drinking plenty of water throughout the day.
- Limit sugary beverages and opt for water, herbal teas, or infused water with fruits and herbs for flavor.

7. **Monitor Blood Sugar Levels:**

- Monitor your blood sugar levels regularly, especially after meals, to assess how different foods affect your blood sugar levels.
- Adjust your meal choices and portion sizes based on your blood sugar readings to maintain stable blood sugar levels.

By understanding macronutrients, practicing portion control, including a variety of foods, balancing your plate, considering meal timing and frequency, staying hydrated, and monitoring blood sugar levels, you can create balanced meals that support your overall health and well-being, including blood sugar control for individuals with diabetes.

Smart Grocery Shopping Tips for Diabetes-Friendly Foods

Smart grocery shopping is essential for individuals with diabetes to maintain a healthy diet and manage blood sugar levels effectively. Here are detailed tips for smart grocery shopping for diabetes-friendly foods:

1. **Plan Ahead:**

- Create a weekly meal plan before heading to the grocery store. Plan balanced meals that include a variety of nutrient-dense foods, such as fruits, vegetables, whole grains, lean proteins, and healthy fats.
- Check your pantry and refrigerator to see what ingredients you already have and make a list of items you need to buy.

2. **Focus on Whole Foods:**

Choose whole, unprocessed foods as much as possible. Opt for fresh fruits and vegetables, whole grains, lean proteins, and healthy fats.

- Limit processed and packaged foods that are high in added sugars, refined carbohydrates, unhealthy fats, and sodium.

3. **Read Food Labels:**

- Pay attention to food labels and ingredient lists. Look for foods that are low in added sugars, saturated fats, and sodium.
- Choose products with minimal ingredients and avoid those with long lists of additives and preservatives.

4. **Choose Low-Glycemic Foods:**

- Select foods with a low glycemic index (GI) to help manage blood sugar levels. Low-GI foods include non-starchy vegetables, whole grains, legumes, and some fruits.
- Avoid high-GI foods such as sugary drinks, processed snacks, white bread, and sugary cereals, which can cause rapid spikes in blood sugar levels.

5. **Incorporate Fruits and Vegetables:**

- Fill your cart with a variety of colorful fruits and vegetables. Choose fresh, frozen, or canned options without added sugars or sauces.
- Aim to include a rainbow of colors to maximize nutrient intake and provide a variety of vitamins, minerals, and antioxidants.

6. Choose Whole Grains:

Opt for whole grains like brown rice, quinoa, whole wheat bread, oats, and barley. These grains are rich in fiber and nutrients and have a lower impact on blood sugar levels compared to refined grains.

7. Select Lean Proteins:

- Choose lean sources of protein such as poultry, fish, tofu, tempeh, legumes, and low-fat dairy products.
- Limit red and processed meats, which are higher in saturated fats and may increase the risk of heart disease.

8. Include Healthy Fats:

- Incorporate sources of healthy fats such as avocados, nuts, seeds, olive oil, and fatty fish like salmon and mackerel.
- Limit saturated and trans fats found in processed foods, fried foods, and baked goods, as they can increase cholesterol levels and raise the risk of heart disease.

9. Be Mindful of Portions:

- Practice portion control when buying foods, especially carbohydrate-rich foods like grains, fruits, and starchy vegetables.
- Use measuring cups, spoons, or visual cues to estimate portion sizes and avoid overeating.

10. Stock up on Healthy Snacks:

- Choose diabetes-friendly snacks like raw nuts, seeds, Greek yogurt, fresh fruit, vegetables with hummus, or whole-grain crackers with cheese.
- Avoid sugary snacks, chips, cookies, and other processed snacks that are high in added sugars and unhealthy fats.

11. Stay Hydrated:

Drink plenty of water throughout the day. Opt for water, herbal teas, or infused water with fruits and herbs instead of sugary beverages.

12. Be Flexible:

Be open to trying new foods and recipes. Experiment with different flavors and cooking methods to keep your meals interesting and enjoyable.

By planning ahead, focusing on whole foods, reading food labels, choosing low-GI foods, incorporating fruits and vegetables, selecting whole grains and lean proteins, including healthy fats, practicing portion control, stocking up on healthy snacks, staying hydrated, and being flexible with your choices, you can make smart grocery shopping decisions that support your diabetes management and overall health.

Portion Control Strategies

Portion control is crucial for individuals with diabetes to manage blood sugar levels, maintain a healthy weight, and promote overall well-being. Here are detailed strategies for practicing portion control:

1. **Use Measuring Tools:**

   - Use measuring cups, spoons, and a kitchen scale to accurately measure portions of food.
   - Become familiar with standard serving sizes for common foods like grains, proteins, fruits, vegetables, and fats.

2. **Visualize Portions:**

   - Learn to estimate portion sizes using visual cues. For example, a serving of meat should be about the size of a deck of cards, a serving of grains should be about the size of a tennis ball, and a serving of cheese should be about the size of a pair of dice.
   - Use everyday objects as references to visualize portion sizes, such as a fist for a serving of vegetables or a palm for a serving of protein.

3. **Plate Method:**

   - Use the plate method to build balanced meals. Fill half of your plate with non-starchy vegetables, one-quarter with lean protein, and one-quarter with whole grains or starchy vegetables.
   - This method helps control portion sizes while ensuring a balanced intake of nutrients.

4. **Half-Plate Rule:**

Apply the half-plate rule when dining out or eating at home. Fill half of your plate with vegetables, one-quarter with lean protein, and one-quarter with whole grains or starchy vegetables.

5. **Pre-Portion Snacks:**

   - Pre-portion snacks into individual servings to prevent overeating. Divide snacks like nuts, trail mix, or popcorn into small containers or bags for easy grab-and-go options.
   - This helps control portion sizes and prevents mindless snacking.

6. **Practice Mindful Eating:**

- eating Pay attention to hunger and fullness cues. Eat slowly, savoring each bite, and stop when you feel satisfied, not overly full.
- Avoid distractions like watching TV or using electronic devices while eating, as this can lead to overeating.

7. **Read Food Labels:**

- Read food labels to understand portion sizes and servings per container. Pay attention to the serving size listed on the label and compare it to the portion you consume.
- Be mindful of hidden sources of added sugars, unhealthy fats, and sodium in packaged foods.

8. **Share Meals:**

When dining out, consider sharing meals with a friend or family member. Many restaurant portions are oversized, and sharing can help control portion sizes and reduce calorie intake.

9. **Use Smaller Plates and Bowls:**

Use smaller plates and bowls to control portion sizes. Research shows that using smaller dishware can lead to smaller portion sizes and reduced calorie intake without feeling deprived.

10. **Be Mindful of Liquid Calories:**

Be mindful of liquid calories from beverages like sugary drinks, alcohol, and fruit juices. Opt for water, herbal teas, or infused water with fruits and herbs to stay hydrated without adding extra calories.

11. **Listen to Your Body:**

Listen to your body's hunger and fullness cues. Eat when you're hungry and stop when you're satisfied, rather than finishing everything on your plate out of habit or obligation.

12. **Plan Ahead:**

Plan meals and snacks in advance to avoid impulse eating and make healthier choices. Pack healthy snacks when you're on the go to prevent reaching for unhealthy options when hunger strikes.

By implementing these portion control strategies, individuals with diabetes can effectively manage their portion sizes, control calorie intake, and improve blood sugar management while enjoying a balanced and satisfying diet.

Tips for Dining Out with Diabetes

Dining out can present challenges for individuals with diabetes, but with proper planning and smart choices, it's possible to enjoy meals while managing blood sugar levels effectively. Here are detailed tips for dining out with diabetes:

1. **Plan Ahead:**

   - Research restaurant options in advance and review their menus online. Look for restaurants that offer a variety of healthy and diabetes-friendly options.
   - Consider calling ahead to inquire about menu options, special dietary accommodations, or ingredient substitutions if needed.

2. **Choose Restaurants Wisely:**

   - Select restaurants that offer healthier options like grilled or baked dishes, salads, and vegetable-based dishes.
   - Opt for restaurants that allow customization of dishes to meet your dietary preferences and needs.

3. **Check the Menu Carefully:**

   - Look for menu items that are lower in carbohydrates, saturated fats, and added sugars. Choose dishes that include lean proteins, vegetables, and whole grains.
   - Be cautious of hidden sources of added sugars and unhealthy fats in sauces, dressings, and marinades.

4. **Control Portion Sizes:**

   - Be mindful of portion sizes, which can be larger than recommended when dining out. Consider sharing entrees with a dining companion or asking for a half portion.
   - Request a to-go container when your meal is served and portion out an appropriate serving size before you start eating to avoid overeating.

5. **Customize Your Order:**

   - Don't hesitate to customize your order to meet your dietary needs. Ask for sauces, dressings, and condiments on the side to control portions and reduce added sugars and unhealthy fats.
   - Request substitutions or modifications to make dishes healthier, such as swapping fries for a side salad or steamed vegetables.

6. **Opt for Grilled or Baked Options:**

   - Choose grilled, baked, or roasted dishes instead of fried options, which tend to be higher in unhealthy fats and calories.

- Look for dishes that are prepared with minimal added oils or butter.

7. **Be Mindful of Sides and Extras:**

- Be cautious of high-carbohydrate sides like bread, rice, potatoes, and pasta. Consider asking for substitutions like extra vegetables or a side salad.
- Limit or avoid high-calorie extras like appetizers, bread baskets, and desserts.

8. **Control Beverage Choices:**

- Opt for water, unsweetened tea, or sparkling water instead of sugary drinks, sodas, and alcoholic beverages.
- Be mindful of portion sizes for alcoholic beverages, and consider lighter options like wine or light beer.

9. **Practice Portion Control with Desserts:**

- If you choose to indulge in dessert, practice portion control by sharing with others or asking for a smaller portion.
- Look for lighter dessert options like fresh fruit, sorbet, or a small serving of dark chocolate.

10. **Monitor Blood Sugar Levels:**

- Monitor your blood sugar levels before and after dining out to assess how different foods affect your blood sugar levels.
- Adjust your meal choices and portion sizes based on your blood sugar readings to maintain stable blood sugar levels.

11. **Stay Active:**

Incorporate physical activity into your day, such as taking a walk after a meal, to help manage blood sugar levels and aid digestion.

By following these tips and making informed choices when dining out, individuals with diabetes can enjoy meals at restaurants while managing their blood sugar levels effectively and promoting overall health and well-being.

Appendix

Glossary of Key Terms

Creating a glossary of key terms related to diabetes can be helpful for individuals looking to understand the terminology associated with the condition. Here's a detailed discussion of key terms:

1. **Blood Glucose (Blood Sugar):**
7. Blood glucose refers to the amount of sugar (glucose) present in the bloodstream. It is the primary source of energy for cells in the body and must be maintained within a certain range for optimal health.
2. **Type 1 Diabetes:**
8. Type 1 diabetes is a chronic autoimmune condition in which the body's immune system attacks and destroys insulin-producing beta cells in the pancreas. This results in little to no insulin production, leading to high blood sugar levels.
3. **Type 2 Diabetes:**
9. Type 2 diabetes is a metabolic disorder characterized by insulin resistance, where the body's cells do not respond effectively to insulin. This leads to high blood sugar levels due to insufficient insulin production or improper insulin utilization.
4. **Insulin:**
10. Insulin is a hormone produced by the pancreas that helps regulate blood sugar levels by facilitating the uptake of glucose from the bloodstream into cells. In individuals with diabetes, insulin may be administered through injections or insulin pumps to manage blood sugar levels.
5. **Insulin Resistance:**
11. Insulin resistance is a condition in which the body's cells become less responsive to the effects of insulin, leading to elevated blood sugar levels. It is commonly associated with type 2 diabetes but can also occur in individuals with obesity, metabolic syndrome, and other conditions.
6. **Hemoglobin A1c (HbA1c):**
12. Hemoglobin A1c, often referred to as HbA1c or simply A1c, is a measure of average blood glucose levels over the past 2-3 months. It is used as a marker of long-term blood sugar control in individuals with diabetes, with lower levels indicating better glucose management.
7. **Hyperglycemia:**
13. Hyperglycemia refers to high blood sugar levels, typically defined as a blood glucose level above the normal range. It can occur in individuals with diabetes due to insufficient insulin production or improper insulin utilization.
8. **Hypoglycemia:**

14. Hypoglycemia refers to low blood sugar levels, typically defined as a blood glucose level below the normal range. It can occur in individuals with diabetes who take insulin or certain medications that lower blood sugar levels.

9. **Carbohydrates:**

15. Carbohydrates are one of the three main macronutrients found in food and beverages, along with protein and fat. They are broken down into glucose during digestion and have the most significant impact on blood sugar levels in individuals with diabetes.

10. **Glycemic Index (GI):**

16. The glycemic index (GI) is a measure of how quickly carbohydrates in food raise blood sugar levels after consumption. Foods with a high GI cause a rapid increase in blood glucose levels, while those with a low GI result in a slower and more gradual increase.

11. **Ketones:**

17. Ketones are chemicals produced by the liver when the body breaks down fat for energy in the absence of sufficient insulin. High levels of ketones can occur in individuals with uncontrolled diabetes, particularly in type 1 diabetes, and may lead to diabetic ketoacidosis (DKA), a serious and potentially life-threatening condition.

12. **Metabolic Syndrome:**

18. Metabolic syndrome is a cluster of conditions that occur together, including high blood pressure, high blood sugar levels, excess abdominal fat, and abnormal cholesterol or triglyceride levels. It increases the risk of developing type 2 diabetes, heart disease, and stroke.

13. **Neuropathy:**

19. Neuropathy refers to nerve damage that can occur in individuals with diabetes, particularly in the hands and feet. It can cause symptoms such as numbness, tingling, pain, and weakness, and may lead to complications like diabetic neuropathy.

14. **Retinopathy:**

20. Retinopathy is a complication of diabetes that affects the blood vessels in the retina, the light-sensitive tissue at the back of the eye. It can cause vision problems, including blurred vision, floaters, and eventually, blindness if left untreated.

15. **Nephropathy:**

21. Nephropathy, also known as diabetic kidney disease, is a complication of diabetes that affects the kidneys. It can lead to kidney damage and impaired kidney function, ultimately progressing to kidney failure if not managed properly.

16. **Polyuria, Polydipsia, Polyphagia:**

22. Polyuria refers to excessive urination, polydipsia refers to excessive thirst, and polyphagia refers to excessive hunger. These symptoms may occur in individuals with diabetes, particularly when blood sugar levels are elevated.

17. **Diabetic Ketoacidosis (DKA)** - Diabetic ketoacidosis (DK)

Nutritional Information for Recipes

Providing detailed nutritional information for recipes is essential, especially for individuals with specific dietary requirements or health conditions like diabetes. Here's a comprehensive discussion of nutritional information for recipes:

1. **Calories:**

Calories represent the energy content of a food or recipe and are measured in kilocalories (kcal) or kilojoules (kJ). It's important to include the total calorie count per serving to help individuals manage their daily calorie intake.

2. **Macronutrients:**

Macronutrients include carbohydrates, proteins, and fats, which are essential for the body's energy needs and overall function. Providing the breakdown of macronutrients helps individuals understand the nutritional composition of the recipe.

a. **Carbohydrates:**

Carbohydrates are the body's primary source of energy and are found in foods like grains, fruits, vegetables, and legumes. Including the total grams of carbohydrates per serving is crucial for individuals with diabetes to manage their blood sugar levels.

b. **Proteins:**

Proteins are essential for building and repairing tissues, as well as supporting immune function and hormone production. Including the total grams of protein per serving helps individuals meet their protein needs and maintain muscle mass.

c. **Fats:**

Fats are important for providing energy, supporting cell growth, and absorbing certain vitamins. Including the total grams of fat per serving, as well as the breakdown of saturated, unsaturated, and trans fats, helps individuals make informed choices about their fat intake.

3. **Fiber:**

Fiber is a type of carbohydrate that the body cannot digest. It helps regulate digestion, stabilize blood sugar levels, and promote feelings of fullness. Including the total grams of fiber per serving helps individuals meet their daily fiber needs.

4. **Sugars:**

Sugars are simple carbohydrates found naturally in foods like fruits and dairy products, as well as added sugars found in processed foods and beverages. Including the total grams of sugars per serving helps individuals monitor their sugar intake, particularly those with diabetes.

5. **Sodium:**

Sodium is a mineral found in salt and is essential for fluid balance, nerve function, and muscle contraction. However, excessive sodium intake can increase the risk of high blood pressure and heart disease. Including the total milligrams of sodium per serving helps individuals limit their sodium intake.

6. **Vitamins and Minerals:**

Vitamins and minerals are essential nutrients that support various bodily functions, including immune function, bone health, and metabolism. Including the percentage of the recommended daily intake (RDI) or daily value (DV) for vitamins and minerals per serving helps individuals ensure they are meeting their nutritional needs.

7. **Allergen Information:**

Including allergen information for recipes helps individuals with food allergies or intolerances identify potential allergens and make safe food choices. Common allergens include nuts, dairy, eggs, soy, wheat, and shellfish.

8. **Serving Size:**

Providing the serving size for the recipe is essential for accurately calculating the nutritional information per serving. It helps individuals portion their food appropriately and track their nutrient intake.

9. **Nutritional Analysis Tools:**

Utilizing nutritional analysis tools or software can help accurately calculate the nutritional information for recipes based on the ingredients used. These tools take into account the nutrient content of each ingredient and provide a comprehensive breakdown of the recipe's nutritional composition.

By providing detailed nutritional information for recipes, individuals can make informed choices about their food intake, monitor their nutrient intake, and manage their health effectively, especially for those with specific dietary requirements or health conditions like diabetes.

Conversion Charts for Ingredients

Conversion charts for ingredients are valuable tools that help individuals accurately measure and substitute ingredients in recipes. Here's a detailed discussion of conversion charts for various ingredients:

1. **Dry Ingredients**:

Conversion charts for dry ingredients typically include measurements in both volume (e.g., cups, tablespoons, teaspoons) and weight (e.g., ounces, grams). This is important because different dry ingredients have varying densities, so measuring by weight can ensure accuracy, especially in baking.

Common dry ingredient conversions:

- 1 cup flour = 120 grams
- 1 cup sugar = 200 grams
- 1 cup oats = 90 grams
- 1 cup nuts = 150 grams

2. **Liquid Ingredients:**

- Conversion charts for liquid ingredients usually include measurements in volume (e.g., cups, fluid ounces, milliliters). These measurements are crucial for accurately measuring liquids like water, milk, oil, and broth.
- Common liquid ingredient conversions:
- 1 cup water = 8 fluid ounces = 240 milliliters
- 1 cup milk = 8 fluid ounces = 240 milliliters
- 1 tablespoon = 0.5 fluid ounces = 15 milliliters
- 1 teaspoon = 0.17 fluid ounces = 5 milliliters

3. **Butter and Margarine:**

- Butter and margarine are often measured by volume (e.g., tablespoons, teaspoons) or by weight (e.g., ounces, grams). Conversion charts for butter and margarine help individuals accurately measure and substitute these fats in recipes.
- Common butter and margarine conversions:
- 1 stick of butter = 8 tablespoons = 4 ounces = 113 grams
- 1 tablespoon of butter = 14 grams
- 1 cup of butter = 16 tablespoons = 8 ounces = 227 grams

4. **Eggs:**

- Eggs are usually measured by quantity rather than weight or volume. However, conversion charts for eggs may provide information on substituting whole eggs, egg whites, or egg yolks in recipes.
- Common egg conversions:
- 1 large egg = approximately 50 grams
- 1 egg white = approximately 30 grams
- 1 egg yolk = approximately 18 grams

5. **Yeast:**

- Yeast is often measured by weight (e.g., ounces, grams) rather than volume due to its active nature. Conversion charts for yeast help individuals accurately measure and use this ingredient in baking recipes.
- Common yeast conversions:
- 1 packet of active dry yeast = 7 grams = 2 ¼ teaspoons
- 1 tablespoon of active dry yeast = 11 grams

6. **Flavorings and Spices:**

- Conversion charts for flavorings and spices typically include measurements in both volume (e.g., teaspoons, tablespoons) and weight (e.g., ounces, grams). This ensures accuracy when using these ingredients in recipes.
- Common flavoring and spice conversions:
- 1 teaspoon = 5 milliliters = 5 grams
- 1 tablespoon = 15 milliliters = 15 grams

7. **Temperature:**

- Conversion charts for temperature help individuals convert between Fahrenheit and Celsius, which is useful for baking and cooking.
- Common temperature conversions:
- Fahrenheit to Celsius: (°F − 32) x 5/9
- Celsius to Fahrenheit: (°C x 9/5) + 32

8. **Other Ingredients:**

Conversion charts may also include measurements for other ingredients like fruits, vegetables, grains, and dairy products. These charts help individuals accurately measure and substitute these ingredients in recipes.

By using conversion charts for ingredients, individuals can ensure accuracy and consistency when cooking and baking, leading to successful and delicious results in the kitchen.

Resources for Further Reading and Support

Resources for further reading and support play a crucial role in providing individuals with diabetes access to reliable information, guidance, and support networks. Here's a detailed discussion of resources available for individuals with diabetes:

1. **Diabetes Organizations and Associations:**

Diabetes organizations and associations provide valuable resources, educational materials, and support networks for individuals with diabetes and their families. Examples include:

- American Diabetes Association (ADA)
- International Diabetes Federation (IDF)
- Juvenile Diabetes Research Foundation (JDRF)
- Diabetes UK
- Canadian Diabetes Association

2. **Websites and Online Platforms:**

Websites and online platforms dedicated to diabetes offer a wealth of information, including articles, blogs, recipes, forums, and support groups. Some reputable websites include:

- Diabetes.org (American Diabetes Association)
- Diabetes.co.uk (Diabetes UK)
- Mayo Clinic Diabetes Center
- WebMD Diabetes Center
- Healthline Diabetes Center

3. **Books and Publications:**

Books and publications written by healthcare professionals, researchers, and individuals with diabetes provide in-depth information on various aspects of diabetes management, including nutrition, exercise, medication, and emotional well-being. Some recommended books include:

- "Think Like a Pancreas" by Gary Scheiner
- "The Diabetes Code" by Dr. Jason Fung
- "Bright Spots & Landmines" by Adam Brown
- "The End of Diabetes" by Dr. Joel Fuhrman
- "Diabetes Burnout" by William H. Polonsky

4. **Medical Journals and Research Papers:**

Medical journals and research papers offer up-to-date information on the latest advancements in diabetes research, treatment options, and management strategies. Access to medical journals may require a subscription or membership to professional organizations. Some reputable journals include:

- Diabetes Care
- Diabetes
- The Lancet Diabetes & Endocrinology
- Journal of Diabetes Research
- Diabetologia

5. Apps and Digital Tools:

Mobile apps and digital tools designed for diabetes management offer features such as blood glucose tracking, meal planning, medication reminders, and educational resources. Some popular apps include:

- MySugr
- Glucose Buddy
- One Drop
- MyFitnessPal
- Fooducate

6. Local Support Groups:

Local support groups and community organizations provide opportunities for individuals with diabetes to connect with others facing similar challenges, share experiences, and receive emotional support. These groups may be facilitated by healthcare professionals, diabetes educators, or peer volunteers.

7. Telemedicine and Virtual Care:

Telemedicine and virtual care services allow individuals with diabetes to consult with healthcare professionals remotely, receive medical advice, and access diabetes management support from the comfort of their homes. These services may include virtual consultations with endocrinologists, diabetes educators, dietitians, and psychologists.

8. Social Media and Online Communities:

Social media platforms and online communities dedicated to diabetes provide a platform for individuals to connect, share experiences, ask questions, and offer support to one another. Popular platforms include Facebook groups, Twitter chats, Instagram accounts, and online forums like TuDiabetes and Diabetes Daily.

By utilizing resources for further reading and support, individuals with diabetes can empower themselves with knowledge, connect with supportive communities, and effectively manage their condition to improve their overall health and well-being.

Thank you for chosen this Diabetic Diet Cookbook for Beginners 2024! Your support fuels my passion for healthy cooking.